SPORTS
WITHOUT
PRESSURE

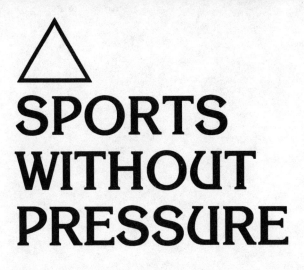

SPORTS WITHOUT PRESSURE

A GUIDE FOR PARENTS & COACHES OF YOUNG ATHLETES

By Eric Margenau, Ph.D.

GARDNER PRESS, INC.
New York △ Sydney △ London

Library of Congress Cataloging-in-Publication Data
Margenau, Eric
    Sports without pressure.

    1. Sports for children—Psychological aspects.
I. Title.
GV709.2.M33   1989   796'.019'22   89-16998

Book Design by Raymond Solomon

This is lovingly dedicated to my children,
DANIELLE and MAX,
who provide a living laboratory
for many of the concepts presented herein
and to my wife, ANNE,
who applies them far more expertly than I.

Acknowledgments

When I first began work on this book, it centered on the portion of an athlete's career that involves a transition from athlete to private citizen. Having had to forfeit the possibility of an athletic career to a knee injury in my last year of college, I am familiar with the despair that can strike when an athlete reaches the end of the line. It was my agent, Jay Acton, who lent me the insight and literary guidance that ultimately led to the book being expanded to include the full developmental span of the athlete's life. It was his vision of what this book should be that resulted in its present scope and form.

After settling on the book's shape, it was left to the expertise of Ardy Freidberg, a man capable of taking my thoughts and concepts as well as the many case histories and forging them into a comprehensive reflection of my point of view. This he did with a facility that was enjoyable to observe. The give and take that we shared was as gratifying in many respects as was seeing the final results.

Finally, gratitude goes to my editor and publisher, Gardner Spungin, who patiently and expertly shepherded the manuscript through the process of becoming a book. This can be an agonizing time, but in his hands the experience seemed nearly painless.

In conclusion, the opportunity to do this book with these close friends, as well as having my wife, a skillful therapist in her own right, review and comment on my book has made the experience of sharing my thoughts and ideas challenging and rewarding, but most of all fun.

Contents

△ △

Introduction

THE MESSAGES OF *Sports Without Pressure* are simple though the implementation of the principles I'm going to present are a bit more difficult. The first message is: Provide your child with a sports experience regardless of how you personally feel about the importance of sports in life. The second message is more general: Step back and take a good look at yourself as a parent and at the way you relate to your child and his or her sports experience. In many ways this second parental task couldn't be easier. In many other ways it couldn't be harder.

Of course, the concept of taking a good look at your relationship with your child can apply equally to any of the myriad aspects of parenting, but this book focuses on only one of those aspects—the sports experience.

To some parents, especially those who are not athletically inclined, this sports experience may seem like one of the less important parental responsibilities, but research in the field and my twenty years of experience as a practicing psychologist have convinced me that an early and frequent exposure to sports produces children who are healthier both physically and emotionally, and who grow up to become healthier adults.

△

James Michener, in his landmark book *Sports in America*, says it very well. In a chapter extolling the virtues of athletics for children, he says:

> I believe that children, like little animals, require play and competition in order to develop. I believe that play is a major agency in civilizing infants. I believe that big-muscle movement helps the infant establish his balance within the space in which he will henceforth operate. I believe that competition, reasonably supervised, is essential to the full maturing of the individual.

I can't state the case any more clearly or more eloquently. Though I'm quite certain Michener was writing from his own observations and not from a thorough study of the field, his points are precisely on the mark from both a physical and a psychological point of view. Play is not only natural among humans and animals but it is a necessity for natural, normal, and complete development. A number of studies have shown that children who play frequently with other children or with adults tend to socialize and adjust better as adolescents and adults.

Muscle movement creates body awareness, which gives a child a sense of space and spatial relationships. This sense of knowing your body, how much space it takes, and how it moves through space is important physically and emotionally because it gives a child a sense of self-assurance and control.

Healthy competition provides a natural, nonthreatening emotional outlet for children. Even a seemingly noncompetitive game like hide-and-seek has its competitive ingredients, and this kind of competition should be encouraged rather than stifled.

On the other hand, competition among children should not be forced, exaggerated, or overemphasized by adults. Overemphasis, even for those children who show exceptional athletic skills at an early age, is not healthy. That's what this book is all about.

Throughout *Sports Without Pressure* I will continue to make these main points in various ways:

1. An athletic experience is not only good, but it is *essential for all children*, not just children of parents who are interested in sports.

2. Sports—like books, music, and art—are one of life's important growth experiences and parent and child will both grow together in the experience.

3. Sports are fun and should be kept fun.

4. Competition is fine, but it should be kept friendly with the emphasis on participation rather than outcome.

5. Parents should not pressure a child to excel, regardless of that child's abilities.

6. An interest in sports can lead in two directions—one is recreational and amateur in nature and the other is professional. Either of these outcomes can be productive physically and emotionally throughout life.

The pressure referred to throughout this book takes many forms, but in essence I'm talking about the pressure parents put on their children to perform excellently and compete successfully in sports. It's the kind of pressure—often applied subtly and or even unconsciously—that says quite clearly to a child that performance is more important than participation, winning is more important than how you play the game, and, in fact, that there is nothing wrong with winning at all costs.

The implication of this pressure to excel is that games are work, not fun. This is the antithesis of what games, especially games for children, are all about and the results of this heavy and constant pressure can have disastrous short- and long-term results.

Perhaps the classic case that illustrates this point is that of Andrea Jeager, the tennis player whose career flowered so quickly and brilliantly in the early 1980s when she was just barely in her teens and wilted so rapidly when she became a young adult. For Jeager, it was not a case of deteriorating skills—she was too young for that—but a combination of accumulated pressure and what we've come to call "burnout" that ended her playing days prematurely.

Jeager had trained for a career in tennis from the time she was old enough to hold a racket. It was immediately apparent that she had a marvelous talent for the game and took instruction very well. She quickly moved through the amateur ranks and she went on to become the youngest pro on the women's tennis tour. She did extremely well during her brief career and at the tender age of sixteen she was ranked number three among all the women tennis players in the world.

But at age eighteen she reached a point where she mentally gave in to the constant pressures of tour competition and stardom. Quite suddenly, she decided to give up her tennis and her six-figure income to become, as she said at the time, "more of a regular person."

The lessons of Andrea Jeager's situation are of the "too much" variety. Jeager started serious training *too* early, she was subjected to *too* much pressure from all sides, she had *too* much coaching *too* early, *too* much exposure to the rigors and adversities of the adult world, *too* much success *too* fast, and *too* much adulation from adults and peers for the average teenager to handle.

Granted, very few athletes reach the pinnacle of their careers at such a young age, but regardless of age, few athletes are emotionally prepared for the demands, both physical and mental, of success in the world of big-time athletics. Today's sports pages are filled with stories of drug abuse and criminal activity by athletes that attest to this fact.

My practice also reveals to me that the pressure to perform is not limited to how well a youngster does on the baseball diamond, the basketball court, or the soccer field. That same kind of pressure to perform is often applied by well-meaning parents who want their child to excel in nursery school, in playing the violin, in dancing, and in art. This kind of pressure very often results in the same kinds of problems Andrea Jeager was faced with in her young life. My point is, much of this emotional destruction can be prevented if parents take the time to get to know their own needs and those of their children.

Throughout this book I'll be using case histories, primarily from my own practice (names changed to protect privacy), to illustrate the points I'm making and to offer lessons that are applicable to all parents whether they have a child who is a gifted athlete or one who simply likes to play the game for fun and exercise.

The first three chapters of *Sports Without Pressure* give background on the role of sports in American society and of athletics and sports in child development. The succeeding chapters are more "how-to" in nature. Through examples, I'll explain when and how to:

▷ Introduce athletics and then sports into your child's life;

▷ Recognize and deal with the natural and unnatural pressure parents put on their children;

▷ Take that parental pressure off;

▷ Approach the fork in the road that occurs at about age eleven when the choice should be made between serious athletic training and sports for health and recreation.

However, although this book focuses on the importance of athletics and sports in the life of a child, it is also about the psychology of child rearing in general. Clearly, there is much here for parents that is broadly applicable to all parent-child relationships, and that is part of the point of and the lessons to be learned from sports participation by both parent and child.

△ Athletics versus Sports △

At an early age athletics and sports are not synonymous so I think it will be helpful to take the time to define the difference between the two terms. For our purposes, the difference is primarily one of the age of the child. In this book I refer to athletics as movement, the type of movement that falls into the category of gross motor activities and body awareness. This type of activity, which doesn't require much conscious thought, includes crawling, walking, climbing, running, jumping, rolling on the floor, and throwing a ball. It doesn't include catching a ball because that requires a more mature development of fine motor control and hand-eye coordination, and this doesn't occur until a child is nearly five years old.

At five, sports and games more naturally become part of a child's life. At that age a child has lost much of his or her baby fat, which makes movement easier, hand-eye coordination has developed sufficiently to judge distances with some accuracy, and the child has developed the intellect and maturity to understand the general principles of games and their rules, and to abide by those rules.

So, athletics or movement are the first steps in the progression and sports and games are the second.

△ Self-Evaluation △

One final point. Throughout this book I'll be discussing, explaining, and illustrating through examples, the psychological importance of sports for children and the psychological implications of sports for the child and the entire family. Self-evaluation is the key to much of what I'll be talking about, so at various points you'll be asked to make these evaluations in order to more fully understand your own feelings and your relationship to your child.

This is sometimes something like looking in the mirror with your clothes off. You'll see a lot of blemishes that you usually don't pay much attention to or which you choose to ignore. But it's not only the blemishes we are looking for here. Positive factors are equally important and valuable measuring sticks. The absolutely crucial issue is that of honesty. You must make these evaluations honestly. You'll only be cheating yourself and your child if you hedge, avoid, or evade the obvious.

1

Sports in American Society

*I*T WOULD BE hard to overestimate the importance of sports in American society. We are an active people, a nation of participants, spectators, bettors, and second-guessers.

▷ An estimated 100 million people of all ages regularly participate in organized and individual sports that range from bowling and softball to swimming and mountain climbing.

▷ Hundreds of millions of people watch live and televised sports events on a regular basis.

▷ Untold billions of dollars are legally and illegally wagered annually on horse races, boxing, football, baseball, and nearly every other sport.

▷ It's a rare conversation that doesn't turn to sports at some point, and true sports fanatics can spend hours replaying, dissecting, and second-guessing every play in yesterday's big game.

This American passion for sports is no more clearly evident than in the news media. Virtually every newspaper of any size has a sports section, though it probably doesn't have a special

section for books, music, or even international news. Every radio
and television news program has a sportscaster who reports on
events of local and national interest. Most major cities have at
least one radio call-in show devoted entirely to sports, and nationally there are several cable TV channels that carry sports events
exclusively. In addition, there are at least seventy-five nationally
distributed weekly and monthly sports publications (not to mention scores of privately published newsletters) that treat every
aspect of the sporting life in exhausting detail. And the summa-
rizing, categorizing, and analyzing of sports statistics is a business all its own.

The total annual revenue generated by sports-related activities in this country, including collegiate athletics, has been estimated conservatively at $20 billion. And the salaries of
professional athletes, which have skyrocketed in the last ten
years, are further evidence of the public's insatiable interest in
watching sports events live and on television.

Even our language has been permeated by sports-related jargon. Such everyday expressions as "out in left field," "game
plan," "ballpark figure," "hard ball," "Monday morning quarter-
back," "roll with the punches," and "feeling up to par," are only
a few of the phrases that have originated in sports and have been
integrated into the vernacular. These expressions are in daily use
from Wall Street to the White House and they are part of the
conversations of doctors, real estate brokers, barbers, house-
wives, and children of all ages. Interestingly, some of the people
who so casually use this sports jargon have only a passing interest in sports and no real idea which sport a particular expression
comes from. But no matter. It's a rare American who doesn't have
an interest in some sport, either as a participant, a spectator, or
a gambler.

This American fascination with sports is nothing new. Histor-
ically, sports have played a large role in our cultural life, though
until this century athletics was the nearly exclusive province of
men and boys. Often the first toy introduced into Johnny's crib
was a ball (Mary was given a doll to play with) and as soon as
he could walk Dad had his son out in the backyard playing catch
and swinging a bat. When Johnny was old enough to play ball
with the other boys in the neighborhood his mother would keep
his dinner warm in the oven until he came home exhausted and
hungry. He was rarely scolded when he stayed out until it was
too dark to see the ball even when it was thrown straight up in

the air. Only young girls, called "tomboys," were included in this "boyish" play and they did so at the risk of taunts from their girl friends and their mothers, who thought they should be acting like little Mary down the street.

Sports remained mostly a man's and boy's world until the 1950s, when the steady growth of leisure time and a burgeoning interest in sports by girls and women brought a dramatic increase in sports participation at all levels by both sexes.

Then, in the mid-1970s the fitness boom hit this country and people who had never seriously considered playing a game or doing formalized exercise got caught up in the frenzy to get fit. When medical findings—the by-products of the jogging and exercise explosion—began to show that regular vigorous physical activity was good for health in general and cardiovascular fitness and weight control in particular, the ranks of the exercisers swelled again. Millions of people, recognizing the significance of these findings, saw the potential rewards of working up a sweat and they too turned to jogging and other exercise as a way of buying insurance for the future.

Running, the easiest and most natural of all athletic movements, quickly became the most popular alternative for those who had only dabbled in exercise and it made instant "athletes" of a whole new group of people who, until they began to run, never thought of themselves as athletes at all. These new converts quickly became "competitors" by entering ten-kilometer races and marathons as if they were strolls around the block. Through their running, many of these people—almost as many women as men—became habitual exercisers who spent almost as much time proselytizing as running. The younger members of this group, who went on to get married and have children, have inculcated their offspring with the same desire for fitness, and this has created a new generation of exercisers and sports fans.

Sports and exercise have reached new highs in participation, and now that all age and sex boundaries have fallen, young and old, men, women, and children alike, are in the gyms, the parks, and the streets pursuing their favorite recreational and fitness activities.

The most popular sports in America today, in the order of the number of participants, are walking, swimming, running, tennis, and golf, but such activities as aerobics, racquetball, soccer, hiking, softball, and bowling are also immensely popular in every part of the country. Even the most conservative estimates put the number of people who actively participate in one sport or another above 50 million. The most optimistic surveys say that 120 million people are involved in some kind of athletic activity on a regular basis, and in this case means three or more times each week.

As the popularity of sports has grown, several new industries devoted to meeting the special needs of exercisers have also developed. The clothing industry responded immediately by providing special clothes, shoes, and other equipment to eager athletes. Today there are special shoes for every sport from walking to mountain climbing and special clothes to go with those shoes. The sporting goods industry has adopted the newest techniques in space age technology and have introduced lightweight racquets for tennis and racquetball, new shafts for golf clubs, and special materials for bicycles, skis, surf boards, and home exercise machines which make them more useful and affordable. The related business of health and fitness clubs has also grown from a specialty service to one that serves hundreds of thousands of members a year, and the vitamin, health food, and diet businesses have skyrocketed.

There are two basic reasons for this national sports mania. The first is physical. Man is a physical animal, made to move, to walk, to run, to jump, but not to sit still. Sports and games provide the kind of physical activity that meets man's basic needs to be active and vital and healthy.

The second reason, and possibly more important, is psychological and emotional. Sports provides both participant and spectator the opportunity to satisfy two important psychological needs that are vital to healthy development—fantasy or escapism, and self-esteem.

Fantasy is a form of escapism that we all engage in from time to time. Fantasy can have a negative effect when carried to extremes, but the natural use of fantasy can be a positive diversion from pressures on the job, at school, or in personal relationships. In short, fantasy is a healthy form of release that allows the mind to wander and wonder.

Sports provides an abundance of fantasy opportunities for spectators and participants alike. As spectators, we can quite easily transport ourselves into a fantasy in which we are part of the action—probably the star of that action—and this boosts our psyches and helps to relieve our anxieties. Like Walter Mitty, whose fantasies took him to the cockpit of a fighter plane and the operating room of a hospital, we can use fantasy as a release from the pressures of reality. This is a healthy process unless it becomes a way of avoiding reality.

As participants, we used fantasy differently. Very few people can play games at the professional level or even the high amateur level, but anyone can put on a pair of running shoes and go out and jog and pretend to be in an important race. Anyone can grab a tennis racket and hit a few with a partner or against a wall and pretend to be in the finals at a big tournament. Anyone can buy a baseball hat and throw the ball around with his son and pretend to be the star pitcher. And in these activities there is that moment, probably only fleeting, when the participant can fantasize that he or she is not just any star but Eammon Coghlan winning the mile at the Millrose Games, Chris Evert serving at match point at Wimbledon, or Roger Clemens striking out the side with his blazing fast ball. These healthy fantasies are readily available in sports and they can be realized anywhere from the backyard basketball court in Kansas City, Missouri, to the dusty ball field in Tyler, Texas.

It's an interesting psychological point that sports fantasies are easier to create than fantasies about being a ballet dancer or a Shakespearean actor. The healthy mind finds it much easier to send the image that you are someone who does the same things you can do in everyday life only better. It's much harder to put yourself in the position of declaiming a soliloquy from *Hamlet* on a Broadway stage than to imagine swinging a bat in the style of Pete Rose. It's easier to visualize yourself as a golfer stroking a perfect putt than as a prima ballerina dancing the lead in *Swan Lake*.

Another reason people have sports-related fantasies is that sports images are more readily available on television. It's almost impossible to spin the television dial and find modern dance at any hour of the day or night, but at almost any hour, twenty-four hours a day, the dial spinner can find a sports event of some kind on television even if it's only a rerun of last season's Super Bowl game.

Fantasy and escape are important psychic elements that sports provide, but the most important psychological reward offered by sports is the opportunity to experience and build self-esteem, to actually go out and do something as well as you can possibly do it, even if that means doing it only adequately. The level of skill displayed is much less important than the act of participation itself.

The link between sports participation and the development of self-esteem is direct. Sports offers the opportunity to at some point (and possibly only one time) execute a single movement perfectly, so perfectly that no star could do it better. If a ten-year-old plays basketball long enough, there is going to be that one sweet moment in time when he's shooting baskets in the driveway just before dinner and imagining himself as Larry Bird of the Boston Celtics. As the clock winds down in his head, that ten-year-old is ready for the last shot with two seconds to go in the championship game. That youngster can sink that shot and go into the house and sit down to dinner feeling just like a sports star. Little in life is quite as sweet as a sports fantasy fulfilled, and there is little that builds self-esteem as well as a sports experience.

The other psychological dynamics that come into play in athletics are:

▷ The identification that comes from belonging to a group and being part of a team;

▷ The satisfaction of peer approval;

▷ The joy of being involved in trying to achieve something your friends are also trying to achieve.

These are all critical elements in the development of the psyche.

Additionally, sports are so important in society because they offer opportunities for the whole family to be involved in an activity, whether it's throwing the Frisbee on the beach or playing touch football in the backyard. Sports gives every family member, regardless of age or ability, the chance to share a common experience. One of the beauties of sports is that it isn't necessary to be completely knowledgeable to express interest. Obviously, detailed knowledge enhances the degree of enjoyment of anything, but that knowledge is not a necessity in sports. Games may sound and look complicated at first glance but there is no sport in which the essence can't be described in one or two sentences and that's simple enough for most everyone to understand.

Finally, no parent should find it hard to utilize a child's interest or participation in sports as a vehicle for establishing better communication with that child. In many families, this is the bridge that gets everyone through the tough times. Sports can be the great equalizer.

The reasons sports are such a large part of American society is that they are physically and psychologically multidimensional and for that reason, they meet human needs on many levels. There are not many activities in life that combine so many physical and psychological elements or are as responsive to so many psychological, emotional, and social needs.

For society in general, sports creates a reason for people to come together, for sharing a communality of experience, for developing self-esteem, and for enriching the inner life through fantasy. What offers a better combination than that?

CHAPTER

2

△   △

Winning Isn't Everything

WANT TO GET laughed out of the room? Next time the issue of sports, children, and competition comes up in the after-dinner conversation just say, "I've always thought that it's not whether you win or lose but how you play the game that counts."

In today's highly competitive, upwardly mobile society that comment is looked on as simplistic or naive at best, ill-informed or ignorant at worst. And I practically guarantee that someone in the group will launch into a lecture about sports as a metaphor for life and point out the "big bucks" to be made in professional sports. This lecture usually ends with a paraphrase of a quote from the late Vince Lombardi who, as coach of the Green Bay Packers pro football team, once said, "Winning isn't everything, it's the only thing."

Vince Lombardi is said to have been a great man in many ways, but I think that single exaggerated statement, so often quoted by sports writers, parents, and even children, has done more to distort the true meaning and value of sports in the minds of people in this country than any other pronouncement about sports and competition. More importantly, Lombardi's credo has been used by misguided and overzealous parents to put the pressure on their children not only to perform well, but to excel at all costs.

This parental pressure has done much to destroy the basic joyful pleasure of sports participation for children. Unfortunately, it often results in a heavy emotional cost to parents and youngsters as well.

This "win at all costs" attitude has been further fueled by the fact that in the last two decades sports has become a multibillion dollar industry in America and winning the game on the field now equates very closely with dollars in the bank for those who are very successful. This fact has been used to justify the application of even more pressure to perform.

You don't have to go any farther than the local Little League park to get a firsthand look at the way this sometimes subtle, sometimes overt, always destructive pressure is applied. You may even have applied a little of it yourself. It begins well before the game with the instructions to "Hit a home run" or "Strike 'em all out." During the game it takes the form of chastening a child (your own or another member of the team) for not getting a hit or for dropping a fly ball, even for making a good, but not perfect, play. And of course, it takes the form of berating the umpire for perceived errors in judgment, harassing the manager to get and keep your child in the game, and at times, it even leads to an embarrassing fist fight with another parent.

Of course, parents don't believe they do and say these things so I often use a videotape camera in my practice to prove the point. While we're discussing the subject in my office, I turn on the camera. Later I play back the tape. There is nothing like the reality of instant replay because it gives the parent a chance to see himself saying some truly terrible things, remarks he would claim he never said except for the proof on the videotape. Parents are shocked and frightened by what they see and their first reaction is, "My God, am I really saying those things about my child? What am I doing?"

How did this happen? How did simple children's games become deadly serious work instead of fun? Why are parents so concerned with winning and losing that they are willing to put their own egos and those of their children on the line? Why do families spend thousands of dollars to send a child to a professional sports camp in the hope that the child will become a big star someday?

Just turn on your television set and you'll find the answer to all of these questions. The inspiration is right there in living color. On any weekend and most weeknights the TV screen is filled with professional and amateur sports events, with "high-fives," with index fingers pointing out that "We're number one," with pomp and slavish adulation, with award ceremonies, with the totaling of prize money to be won or contracts to be signed by the "champions."

Though it rarely does so for youngsters, it's a picture that has inspired unrealistic visions of fame and financial security in the minds of more than one parent, a vision that has prompted parents to launch their children on a serious sports program with little thought given to the effects of such an adventure on the child, the child's siblings, relations between the parents and the child, the relations between parent and parent, and finally, the impact on the family bank account.

Surely any logical person could do the simple mathematics that prove that the dream of achieving financial success in professional sports is more an elaborate fantasy than a realistic possibility. The newly popular sport of gymnastics offers a perfect example of the odds against even the talented athlete. There are only twenty or so spots open for women on the American Olympic gymnastics team and in one famous school alone there are some 2,000 hopefuls practicing, praying, and paying. Add this figure to the number of girls training in other professional schools and on their own with private coaches and the total pool of candidates for those twenty spots is more than 20,000. These are not betting odds. It's much like playing the lottery; everyone has a mathematically slim chance of winning but only one in a million actually wins.

Baseball offers the same incredibly long odds against success. Literally millions of young boys play baseball in the thousands of leagues around the country. Many of these youngsters are good players, some are great, and a very few are truly exceptional. If a boy has professional baseball on his mind (or even winning a college baseball scholarship), he must be one of those truly exceptional players. Setting aside the college scholarship, there are some 650 positions available in major league baseball and of those jobs perhaps ten percent or fifty are open each year. It's not hard to see that even "great" players can get left behind in the scramble for one of these coveted jobs. For those few who make it, the rewards are great.

I work with young athletes (both talented and average) and the parents of these youngsters every day in my practice and I know that very often the true value and meaning of sports participation has been squeezed out by the knowledge that an exceptional athlete can become a millionaire playing a game. I've never yet met a child under twelve who was seriously thinking about becoming a professional athlete, though he or she may give lip service to the idea. But I've met many parents who have that goal in mind for their child even before the child has shown any interest in sports, let alone any particular talent. In that struggle to reach the mythical "pot of gold" at the end of the rainbow, I have seen parents invest their egos and their life savings, and children invest their energy and their childhood in a wrong-headed quest for real gold in which both child and parent suffer severe emotional consequences.

This does not mean that I think that playing sports seriously or for fun is the least bit destructive. Quite the contrary. I think sports are wonderful and I encourage parents to give their children a sports experience as early as possible, regardless of whether the parents have any real interest in sports or not. Physical activity is a vital element in early childhood development and I don't think it can begin too early.

But even as I encourage parents in this direction I also urge them to make those first experiences (and later ones, as well) as much fun as possible. In my practice I try to focus families on the inherent values of athletic participation and away from the desire to "make" a child into an athletic machine. There are those that say sports are a metaphor for life and that children who do well in sports will win in life. But doing well in sports does not correlate at all with winning in life.

I stress the fact that every time a child plays a game the parent is offered a positive parenting opportunity. Each time a child touches a ball the parent can say: "Good catch," "Nice try," "Great," "That's terrific." There is nothing a child can possibly do, including the ultimate failure in sports—striking out—that a parent can't convert into a positive event. It's so easy to say, "Boy, you got up to the plate, you stood in there, you took your cuts and I think you were great." The idea is to reinforce participation and effort, and not to demean "trying" for any reason. This is a rare chance for parents, a genuine "no-lose" situation. So, in fact, sports provides even the most inept child with the opportunity to receive parental approval. What more can we ask.

Unfortunately, parents can turn this positive into a negative quite easily. I've seen a father yell at his son because the boy got a hit, only it was on the ground instead of in the air, and I've seen much worse, including parents slapping their children for not playing up to the parent's standards of excellence. The point is that unqualified support of a child's efforts is crucial and sports provides the opportunities to do this in abundance. Used in this way, sports can be a learning ground for parenting. As a parent learns the importance of a child's participation, there is a carry-over for the parent in the child's other life pursuits. So, in effect, sports trains parents to support, teach, encourage, communicate, and be sensitive to their children.

If parents can avoid the potential pitfalls, athletics can create a wonderful experience for the child and the entire family. So I implore parents to take the pressure off. Resist the urge to turn the athletic field into a classroom. Sports should be fun, warm, exciting, and above all, something to look back on with fond memories. And those positive images are permanent. What isn't important is that your child become a superstar. What is important is that he or she is a healthy child who becomes a healthy adult.

△ *3* △

The Value of Athletics

I BEGAN TO formulate my theories about the psychological value of sports about ten years ago when I was treating an eleven-year-old boy named Jerry. He was originally brought to me by his parents because he was having a variety of adolescent problems that individually were not of much concern but which collectively were distressing to his parents.

In looking over Jerry's medical history I found that he had gone through a three-year period of hormonal changes that alternately resulted in his gaining weight to the point of obesity and then slimming down to a size that was normal for his age. I thought this might have something to do with his problem. I discovered that it did to a certain extent, but not to the degree that it might have if there had not been another important element in his life—sports.

Jerry's parents, both professional people and athletes, told me that from the time Jerry was able to crawl he was encouraged to participate in sports and that they had continued to encourage him to participate even during his heavy periods when he was more awkward. In working with the boy, I quickly realized that his growing-up problems were only passingly related to his weight problem. And the reason for this was that his physical

△

activity had helped him develop a degree of body awareness and
a sense of self which allowed him to continue in his various athletic pursuits and the other activities in his life whether he was
fat or thin.

And beyond athletics, Jerry's positive self-image permitted
him to socialize with his peers both inside and outside of school
and to go about life in general without undue concern about his
physical appearance.

I concluded then, and I've since corroborated the evidence in
my work with other patients, that Jerry's sports history had been
influential in helping him through his periods of overweight and
awkwardness. I'm thoroughly convinced that his problems would
have been worse if he had not been involved in athletics.

The sense of mastery and confidence that comes to a child
from being able to use his or her body in a competent way—
not necessarily in an exceptional way—has long-term emotional
rewards far beyond being able to throw, catch, or kick a ball. Surprisingly, such cases as Jerry's are more typical than unusual.
When a young person is confident of the way he stands, walks,
and runs, that confidence infuses all the other activities in his
life and this confidence continues to be an integral part of the
psyche when the child becomes an adult.

It may be a strong statement to make, but in my opinion, a
parent who says that he or she is not interested in sports and
doesn't value athletics for their child, is acting irresponsibly. This
is not to say that intellectual stimulation is unimportant, only
that physical stimulation is equally important. This means that
the same father who starts reading books to his one-year-old
should also roll the ball back and forth across the floor to his
child, and that the mother who plays classical music for her baby
should also tumble around on the floor with her baby.

The reason I am so firmly committed to the idea is that my
experience in working with children, and with adults as well, has
convinced me beyond a doubt that physical and psychological
development are intimately interrelated. Of course, I'm not the
first to make this connection. There is considerable research on
the subject and most of it supports the close connection between
physical activity and mental health. Recently, some researchers
have successfully used a regimen of running as a treatment for
severe depression and other mental illness, and stretching exercises are being tried with Alzheimer's patients in an attempt to
reverse or slow the effects of that disease on the brain.

Further, I'm convinced, as many psychologists are, that physical movement has a tremendous impact on the development of a child's positive self-image, which is acknowledged to be *the* critical element in human character formation. But even if these studies didn't exist, I'd feel the same way because of my own observations with my patients of the interaction of body movements and the psyche.

Psychologists are not prone to agree on many things, but one thing we do agree on is the importance of a positive self-image to a healthy and active life. And the fact is, there is no more effective way of developing a child's self-image than by the early and frequent exposure of that child to athletic movement and eventually to sports.

Given the evidence, then, the question is not whether sports are good or whether they should be part of a child's life, but how to find the best way to make athletics a part of a child's everyday life and how soon to start.

But before I get to that, a little information about human psychological development will help to explain why the physical— that is, athletic—aspect of a youngster's growth is such a critical matter.

The term *self-image* refers to the *ego,* the word Sigmund Freud used to describe the "I" part of the unconscious mind. In simple terms, the ego, which Freud thought represented one third of the elements that make up the unconscious, is that part which is affected by the environmental or external forces exerted on a child by society in general and by parents in particular. For our purposes, self-image and ego are interchangeable. The terms *self-esteem, self-concept,* and *self-worth* can also be used as synonyms for self-image and all refer to the ego.

Freud called the other two thirds of the unconscious the *id* and the *superego.* The id is the instinctual part of the mind. It is driven by impulses and needs and is the part that is constantly seeking satisfaction for such things as the feelings of hunger and thirst or the need for human warmth, closeness, and reassurance.

The *superego* is governed by things that are learned. Knowing the difference between right and wrong is a function of the *superego.* In essence, it acts as an internal conscience or control center for the ego and it serves to keep the ego under control in mentally healthy people. The *superego* imposes the feeling of guilt a person suffers after spanking his child, or after calling in sick and then spending the day at the beach, or after cheating on his income tax. It's that part of the mind that we'd often like to turn off.

The id and the superego are critically important elements of an individual's mental makeup. But our main concern here is self-image, or ego, a psychological dynamic which amazingly begins to develop even before birth, when the fetus unconsciously picks up a variety of cues and signals from the mother. So, for example, a mother who is worried or has a tough time emotionally during pregnancy is likely to have a child who has assimilated some of her nervousness and uncertainty in utero. This feeling, or emotion, is called anxiety and it actually leaves an imprint on the brain of the child after birth. Of course, a child will pick up a different imprint from a mother who has an easy pregnancy and little other anxiety. These imprints, slight and tenuous at first, become stronger and more permanent toward the end of a pregnancy when the fetus is better formed, but they are constantly being made throughout pregnancy.

Once the baby is born, the mother's easy-going nature or her anxiety is transmitted to the newborn in even more powerful terms. In the broadest sense, those messages indicate to the child that something is right or something is wrong with the way things are going. The baby has no way of knowing what it is that's right or wrong, but he or she picks up the indicative clues through the mother's touch, her movements, and the tone of her voice.

A newborn child, however, is predominantly Id—that is, predominately acting from instinct because it has not yet had time to develop an ego. As the child matures, the ego and superego are layered onto the Id and the three elements act to form the child's character. What's frightening from a parental point of view is that most of this character formation takes place between birth and the age of three. This can be frightening because it leaves so little time for the parent to impart the qualities thought desirable for a normal, happy life.

It's easy to see, therefore, that the environment created for the baby during the early years is critical to the whole future psychological growth and development of the child. In a positive environment free of most stress, a child will develop in a healthy way. The child who grows up in a stressful environment will probably have psychological problems at some point later in life.

At birth and in the first few months of life, a child is in a state that psychologists call primary narcissism. The child makes no

distinction whatever between itself and the rest of the world or
itself and the mother. The child *is* the entire world and the child
views itself, feels itself, as one and the same person as its mother.

At this stage the child is all physical need because it literally
can't survive by itself. It can't walk, talk, get food, or make its
specific needs known in any way (crying indicates a general
need), and if left alone for even a short time—as little as twenty-
four hours—the child will die. So the newborn's primary concern
is survival and it is biologically and psychologically dependent on
the mother for its very existence. This isn't a mystery to the child.
He or she senses that this is the case.

Since the newborn needs the mother's presence, he or she
checks with mother every minute or so when awake. If the
mother leaves the room the child will notice and begin to get
anxious. If the mother's absence lasts for more than a minute or
two, a sense of panic sets in and the baby begins to cry. This
reaction is only instinctual but what the child is essentially saying to itself is, "Wait a minute. I'm supposed to be part of
Mommy. What happened to home base?" Subjected to enough
of this anxiety, uncertainty, and fear (and not all that much is
necessary) the child will develop a permanent feeling of insecurity, a sense of inadequacy, and a subsequent lack of self-esteem
that can last a lifetime.

Obviously, the child is not able to understand exactly what is
happening; his mind only senses that something is wrong. All of
the anxieties are being registered in the unconscious mind and
there is nothing that the child can do to stop it. The facts are
that there is anxiety, fear, anger, and distress in the air and it
is not coming from the child but from the parent or parents or
something in the surroundings.

It takes less than a year for the child to begin to more closely
observe the things that cause anxiety. And unfortunately, the
child not only experiences them but feels responsible for causing
them. This feeling goes back to the fact that in the primary narcissistic state, the child believes it is the only thing that exists in
the world. Therefore, if Mommy is upset, the child must be causing the upset, and if this is true, by definition, there is something
wrong with the child. This causes the child to feel inadequate in
some undefined way and this inadequate feeling registers
unconsciously, etching little lines on the computer chip of the
mind in much the same way as the anxious or tranquil imprints
are made before birth. Only now, by age one, the imprints are
much sharper.

The next step is more serious. In a primary narcissistic state, the message that there is "something wrong" is translated by the child to mean that the child itself is responsible for whatever it is that is wrong. The extension of this is interpreted to mean, "There is something wrong with me" or "They are unhappy because of me" or "What have I done wrong to cause this upset?" The further extension of this is the unconscious thought that, "If I were a better person this would not be happening." These etched marks on the psyche are the foundation of later problems.

In older children who can articulate this guilt feeling, it takes on a specific form. A youngster will say he feels it is his fault that Mommy and Daddy are getting a divorce or that Grandpa died or that his little brother is sick. This is absurd on the face of it but, time after time, youngsters tell me they feel a sense of guilt about just such events and, of course, many events that are of less importance like spilling milk on the table or breaking a toy. Objectively, adults know this can't be the case and will usually tell their children just that. And youngsters themselves sometimes know rationally that they are not the cause of Grandpa's death, but knowing doesn't invalidate the feeling they report.

Between eleven and thirteen months of age, most children enter the period that is called separation or individuation. At this stage the child begins to recognize itself as a being separate from its mother. It can now crawl or walk away and do things on its own like pull pans out of the kitchen cabinets and make noise. It can also put food in its own mouth, and this accomplishment is duly noted by the child as a means of self-preservation. But separation does not mean independence. The child continually checks to make sure the life-support system called Mommy is still around and close enough to help if necessary. Even while individuation is developing, when the support system is missing for a few minutes, if Mommy leaves the room and is out of sight and hearing, the child still becomes extremely anxious.

It's easy to understand then why a baby cries so furiously when the mother leaves the room and why the first time the parents go out and leave the baby with a relative or a babysitter (or even when the mother goes out and leaves the baby alone with the father) the baby will often scream for several minutes and sometimes for hours. It's easy to understand but not easy to accept the fact that the separation has thrown the baby into a state of sheer terror.

As adults we perceive this separation as an absolutely normal thing, but we didn't think it was normal when we were children either. If you try to put yourself in the infant's position, you'll understand that it is quite a different matter. The infant sees its very existence being threatened. It understands simply that Mother is gone, but it can't answer the mind's question, "What am I going to do now?" The baby doesn't have any concept of time and doesn't know if the separation is for five seconds or five hours or forever. What it does know is that its primary life source is absent and, from the infant's viewpoint, that makes the separation a life and death issue.

It is clear that, psychologically, early separation of mother and child for extended periods is not desirable and the ramifications of this separation can have long-term consequences. I know this is at odds with the idea of mothers going to work as soon as physically possible after a baby is born and I personally think this is a question that needs to be closely reevaluated. Mothers have many reasons for going back to work quickly, not the least of which is financial—to bring money into the house. I recognize as well that there is a valid trade-off here. If the mother is unhappy at home and feels her needs are not being met, she will take this out on the child. If it makes the mother happier to go to work and if she feels more fulfilled doing her job, then when she is at home she can give the child more attention and be less resentful.

Note, however, that premature separation clearly does have an affect on children regardless of the mother's motives and the earlier the mother leaves the child the more impact her absence has on the child.

△ MOVEMENT AND SELF-ESTEEM △

That said, where do movement and sports enter into this picture of early childhood development? What does physical movement have to do with developing positive self-esteem, and why? Does movement make positive etchings on the mind's computer chip and what is the value of those etchings?

If you have ever watched your one-year-old child work with the puzzle in which he must put the circles, triangles, and rectangles in the right holes, you have seen part of the answer to the question of whether movement makes a positive imprint on

a child's mind. It may take a matter of days or weeks for the child
to figure out which piece goes where and be able to do the task
with facility, but after the puzzle is conquered the child will continue to work on it. At that point of final learning an older child
will put a puzzle or a toy aside and move on to a new challenge.
But not the very young child. Once the puzzle has been conquered, the one year old sticks with it, doing it over and over
again. Even proud parents can't understand what the fascination
can be after so many successful attempts.

The fascination actually is in the success. The youngster has
developed a physical mastery over the task and each time the
task is completed the child's sense of self-esteem and self-confi-
dence is positively reinforced. There is practically no limit to the
number of times a child will repeat a positive experience.

On the other hand, when a young child is first presented with
a task that is too hard, a real jigsaw puzzle for example, he will
test his abilities once or twice and then leave the puzzle in the
corner for months or perhaps years. The reason? The small child
gets no satisfaction from a negative learning experience. Little
children only learn from positive experiences. The trial and error
method, one of the most important forms of adult learning,
doesn't work well with little children.

This physical development, the ability to accomplish a physical task, reinforces the child's emotional development. In turn,
emotional development reinforces physical development. At the
same time the child is developing this sense of physical mastery,
that is the control over the gross and fine motor coordination and
hand-eye coordination necessary to put a round shape in a round
hole, the child's ego is also developing.

When a child observes that he or she can master something
physical the child experiences what I call the "Ah-ha" dynamic.
The child subconsciously says to itself, "Ah-ha, I can do that."
This is why he or she can do the same puzzle 500 times and
never get tired of it. Each success is a positive boost to the ego
which in turn boosts self-esteem. Each increase in self-esteem
strips away some of the inherent fear of failure and provides the
impetus for the child to attempt more complex physical movements, tasks in which there is likely to be failure in the beginning. This is because the child's healthy self-esteem—gathered
from previous successes—gives it the strength of personality and
the resilience to withstand a failure when it occurs. The realization that his movement can produce an effect, the connection

between the fact that putting a circle in a round hole changes the picture or that pulling on a chain rings a bell, creates a feeling of power in the child which is the basis of the "Ah-ha" dynamic.

With this in mind, it should be easy to see how a diverse set of age-appropriate athletic experiences—not sports *per se*, but simple body movements—develops in the child a level of comfort with his own body which allows him to feel that his body is a good thing, a thing that is within his control, and that it can be made to serve him. The development of self-esteem flows directly from this experience of success and this etches more deeply the groove that signifies competence and mastery into the computer chip of the child's psyche.

These appropriate athletic experiences are within the ability of even the most uncoordinated parent. The most common experience of all is rolling a ball back and forth across the floor. As soon as a child can walk, other movements, from rolling around on the floor to jumping, hopping, climbing, and running, are good for learning body mastery.

As I said, when children are young they learn from success not failure, and that is the true beauty of physical movement. Any physical movement by a child is successful. There is no way it can be a failure, and that successful movement is continuously ego-enhancing. Therefore, every athletic experience *must* be presented to the child as a successful, positive experience. In athletics, it is never necessary to say to a child, "That's wrong," or "Don't do it that way." Since the doing is the important thing, it's simply impossible for anything to be done wrong.

In children and adults, the dominant learning dynamic is imitation and children are great imitators. For this reason, demonstration is the best way to explain something to a child. The demonstration of a movement gives a child the opportunity to create the proper visual image of that movement. If the demonstration is done many times, the child develops a picture in his imagination of how that movement looks and will eventually be able to mimic parts or all of the movement.

So, physical activity has psychological and emotional benefits because it helps a child attain and maintain self-esteem and confidence. The sense of mastery that comes to a child from being able to use his or her body in a competent way—not necessarily in an exceptional way—has long-term emotional rewards apart from athletics. When a young person is confident of the way he or she stands, walks, and runs, that confidence infuses all the other activities in a child's life. And athletics are unique in offering the parent the opportunity to positively reinforce a child's developing feeling of self-esteem in a way that no other activity can.

△ MOVEMENT AND OVERALL DEVELOPMENT △

Now, let's move on to the values of athletics to a child as he or she gets a bit older. What are the basic values of athletics over and above the development of a positive self-image? The answers to these questions are important to every parent regardless of their child's real ability or lack of it.

The values of athletics may begin a bit later in a child's development (at age three or four), but they are worth noting here. A number of studies have shown that athletic activity:

▷ Helps in a child's overall physical development;

▷ Gives a child the opportunity to become familiar with his body and to learn the body's needs and limitations;

▷ Is social as well as physical and teaches a young person how to interact with his or her peers;

▷ Teaches cooperation, teamwork, and how to follow rules;

▷ Helps a child learn for himself if winning or losing is important;

▷ Gives parents the opportunity of offering the child unqualified support;

▷ Helps a child gain acceptance and credibility among his peers.

All of these values are important in the formative years of a child's life and I want to elaborate on each one of them.

Overall physical development. The human body was made to move and the more it moves the better it functions both physically and mentally. There have been many studies of the physical and mental reactions of sedentary people compared to active people at all age levels. These studies show that sedentary children are more often listless and underweight than active children and that a childhood of inactivity may result in serious psychological damage that is irreparable. Sedentary children also may function at a lower mental level as well. On the other hand, active children have been found to be generally more robust, lively, and well-adjusted psychologically as well as more mentally active and alert.

The movements a child makes during an active game or simply when running and jumping require the use of the body's large muscle groups—in the shoulders, back, hips, and legs—and this movement builds, strengthens, and tones muscles. This muscle development is not the kind we think of when we watch a well-developed athlete because the muscles of youngsters don't develop that way, but the movements of athletics do lengthen and strengthen a child's muscles and this is of immediate and long-term value. At the same time, movement stimulates the activity of the brain and causes it to function more rapidly and creatively.

Experiments have shown that this is true regardless of age. People in their sixties and seventies are able to improve their coordination and response time significantly if they exercise on a regular basis. One study showed that a group of sixty-year-olds who exercised three times a week had an equal or better response time when asked to press a button after a light flashed than a group of sedentary twenty-year-old college students.

Unfortunately, even the value of pure physical movement is largely overlooked by parents and schools in this country. The proof of this can be seen in the fact that American youngsters of elementary school age consistently score lower than their counterparts in other industrialized countries around the world on physical fitness tests. Perhaps, now that physical fitness has become a way of life for many adults in America, it is time that we make physical activity a part of the everyday life of our children.

Familiarity with the body. At the same time a child is developing physically through movement, he or she is becoming familiar with the body, how it works, what it can do, what it might be able to do, and what it can't do.

Before the age of three, a child doesn't think consciously about what he is doing but most of the kinesthetic knowledge that is being developed is filed away in the muscles and the brain for future use.

One thing that stands in the way of this accumulation of knowledge is the word *don't*, perhaps the word most often used by parents. For reasons of safety, many parents place limitations on a child's field of movement and this is certainly sensible. This is also where *don't* is a valid response to an active child.

But putting a child in an infant seat or playpen solely for the purposes of control is not a good policy, because both the seat and the playpen drastically restrict movement.

When the child gets a little older and is able to crawl, stand, and then walk, *don't* gets more and more use in most households. The problem is, the use of the word is more often automatic than necessary and parents are unnecessarily restricting the child's movement and preventing the child from becoming more accustomed to its body.

Still later, when the child is taken to the playground, "Don't!" assumes new proportions. It is *the* word on the playground. Certainly, there are times when caution is appropriate but I suspect the caution is more often based on the adult's point of view of the potential danger than on the reality of danger. Besides, cautions and prohibitions have little meaning to a child until he has tested a particular situation for himself. Of course, it may be a bit dangerous to climb on the jungle gym, but in testing himself, a child learns the limits of his physical ability and this is a healthy learning process. This may mean taking a few falls, but so be it.

There are exceptions to a policy of learning from the school of hard knocks, however. Years ago, I was visiting at the home of a friend who was in medical school. The friend and his wife had a one-year-old boy and as we all watched, they allowed him to stand up in his high chair, totter back and forth, and then fall head first onto the floor. Fortunately, he was not hurt, only frightened, but when I asked how in the world they could just let that happen, the mother said, "That's the only way he's going to learn not to stand up in his chair." I told them I thought their attitude was foolish and dangerous, but I don't think my remarks had much impact. At any rate, that's not the sort of freedom of movement I'm talking about here.

Despite my objections to taking needless chances, there is one fact parents, especially first-time parents, don't realize: Children are not nearly as fragile as they seem. It's true that a child's relative clumsiness, the result of a neurological system that is still developing, may get him in some difficult situations, but it is also true that given a bit of time and possibly a little help, the child can usually extricate himself from trouble without serious physical harm.

The overall point here is that using the muscles at an early age builds a sense of knowledge about the body into the unconscious mind of the child and these lessons stay for life.

Interaction and how to relate to other children. The case of Bobby is a good example of how athletics teaches children to relate to each other. When he was first brought to me by his parents at age six, Bobby was not a naturally out-going child and he had only one good friend. He was a little short, though certainly within the normal growth range for his age, but he was also thin and he wore glasses. His parents had no interest whatever in sports; the mother was a college professor and the father a banker. Both parents worked long hours and maintained that they had no time or energy to introduce their son to athletics. Bobby had an older brother and younger sister who were friendly and talkative and all three children were quite bright, but none of them was physically active.

After meeting with Bobby for several weeks, I determined that not only was he underdeveloped physically but also socially. He and I discussed this and he admitted that he liked the idea of participating in sports but he had not received any encouragement from his parents and this made him feel shy and physically inferior to his peers during gym classes at school. He also said that he would like to do something active, something athletic, though he wasn't sure what it was he wanted.

The next time we met I suggested to Bobby that he enroll in a karate class at a private martial arts school near his home. I knew from experience that karate involved physical movement that was relatively simple at the outset and that could be accomplished by a child with little coordination or athletic experience. I also knew that karate classes involved working and sharing with peers. I had made the same suggestion in a number of similar cases in the past and each time the youngster had thrived both physically and socially.

Bobby and his parents accepted my recommendation and he started classes. Almost immediately, I noted (as did his parents) a remarkable change in the boy. In fact, in less than two months he had assumed an entirely new persona. The classes not only gave him an exhilarating physical feeling but raised his level of self-esteem dramatically. Suddenly, he had a feeling that he couldn't be pushed around despite his size and he began fantasizing, in a healthy way, about being a karate expert. At the same time that he was growing in his own mind, he was growing in stature in the eyes of his sister, his brother, and his parents.

And most importantly, and the real reason for suggesting the classes in the first place, was that they gave Bobby a chance to participate in a group activity where effort, not excellence, was rewarded. In the process he made several new friends and has continued to make progress, not only with his lessons, but also in his social life.

I'll talk more about this later, but it's important to remember that the selection of the teacher in any athletic program is hugely important especially for a child with little athletic skill or experience. Take the time to observe the exact class your child will be in, talk with the instructor, and talk with other parents and some of the children in the class. When it comes to teaching athletics to children, there are many inexperienced people and many martinets who are more concerned with enhancing their own egos than in working constructively with children. Most importantly, make sure the class emphasizes activity and participation, not performance. Excellent performance is not what your child is there to achieve.

Certainly, there are other ways a child learns to interact with his peers, but sports activities offer the unique virtue of being natural sources of contact that can occur spontaneously on the streets, at school, and in the gym, or through karate, tennis, swimming, and other classes. Plus, sports offer the type of interaction that is generally rewarding, self-controlling, and nonthreatening.

Cooperation. In a healthy athletic environment, children quickly learn the importance of cooperation. In the most simple situation of all—father and son rolling a ball across the floor to each other—the little game can't take place if one player refuses to cooperate with the other by holding the ball or by continually rolling it so that the other player can't reach it. It doesn't matter if this happens from time to time but if it continues it makes the game impossible to play. This is so easy to understand, such a clear and basic truism, that a child picks it up almost immediately. I'm not saying that a certain amount of teasing and spontaneous fun are the least bit out of order, only that even ball rolling has its conventions and it is those conventions that make the game fun for everyone.

The word *sharing* is vital in the concept of cooperation. But like so many other words we use so casually with children—"be nice," "be gentle," "be polite," "play by the rules"—"sharing" is meaningless in the abstract.

Most parents will remember taking their children to the park to play in the sandbox with the other children from the neighborhood. This is one of the most common parenting experiences, but if you look back on those times you'll recognize that sharing was one of the hardest concepts a child had to learn. Children don't share naturally because from birth, the human instinct is to possess things. And while most parents encourage their children to share a shovel, a pail, or a dump truck, the child doesn't understand the concept and actively resists the idea. In fact, most children give parents a blank' stare when sharing is suggested.

The reason is that a person can't share anything until he is secure about having his own things and knows that he is entitled to them. Sharing simply isn't an organic thing—it's learned. Children can't discriminate "mine" from "yours," because everything is "mine." Yours is mine and mine is mine, but watch out because mine is not yours.

This is one of the psychological elements that carries through in all of life and it's one of the cornerstones of personality—the concept of ownership, possession, sharing, and cooperation.

Athletics helps turn this abstract word into something real because it provides an organic, non-threatening means of integrating the concept of sharing into the personality. A game doesn't impose sharing artificially like parents do in the sandbox. It is something that grows out of the activity itself. The rules of the game enforce the idea. And the real beauty is that sharing in a game is depersonalized and therefore isn't a blow to anyone's ego. Obviously, the concept of sharing and responsibility has many applications outside of sports. From the assembly line to the family camping trip, cooperation is important. And of course this learned sense of cooperation carries over into the games played by older children, teenagers, and adults.

A friend tells this story: As a teenager, he was quite a good golfer, playing competitively for his high school, and playing in public course tournaments in his town. He also liked to play with his father and his father's friends on the weekends and this was where the problem began to develop.

Over the course of several months, Arthur had been steadily improving his scores in rounds played with his peers but for some reason his Sunday morning game was not as good and he began to get more and more irritated with himself. He started to have temper tantrums, to throw clubs, and to curse each time he made a shot that didn't live up to his ever growing expectations. He could see that this was a source of irritation to his father because, though Arthur's anger was directed inward, it was ruining the fun of the game for his father and the rest of the foursome.

Not many Sundays passed before the situation reached a head. Arthur made a bad shot, threw a club, and nearly hit a stranger in the next fairway. At that point his father walked up to him and calmly, but firmly, told him that if he so much as dropped a club in the future, he would never play golf with his son again. This immediately brought home the stupidity and repugnance of his attitude and Arthur apologized to everyone involved, especially his father.

He has continued to play golf all his life and he has never had a serious outburst of temper since that day nearly thirty-five years ago.

Arthur's story illustrates the point that cooperation, a spirit of helpfulness, and a positive approach make sports more fun, but it also makes the point that sports teaches what cooperation is all about. Again, there are many ways to learn how to cooperate and about cooperation, but athletics and sports offers these opportunities many times within a single event, even an event as small as rolling the ball back and forth across the floor.

Teamwork: Teamwork is an extension of cooperation and it applies more to organized games where there are teams, where real rules apply, and where a group of people or players is involved on each side.

Teamwork is a vital element of team sports because the efforts of one person, no matter how dramatic, are not usually sufficient to carry the entire group. I'm not talking here about winning and losing, only about playing the game so that it is fun for all the participants. So what is simply cooperation in small group activities becomes teamwork where it is not possible to accomplish something by yourself.

Basketball, a team sport with only five players on a side, is a perfect example of the necessity for teamwork. One player may score many points in a single basketball game but there is no way he could score those points without the assistance of his teammates and there is no way he could score enough points to win the game by himself. Every player knows this when he goes into the game and every youngster learns this lesson—in a natural way—the first time he plays.

Rules: All games have rules, and the game of life has rules as well. When children first begin to play games the rules are irrelevant. Besides, a young child can easily be confused and frustrated by rules that make no sense in the abstract and are inappropriate in practice. Let me give you an example.

When my daughter was about four years old she asked to go out with me to play tennis. I was delighted with the idea and the next Saturday morning I took her to a sporting goods store to buy an inexpensive, child-sized racquet that she could handle. When we got out to the courts she immediately took the racquet in both hands and held it cross-handed as well. She was ready to go. At that point I could have corrected her grip, but as far as I was concerned any way she could comfortably hold the racquet in her small hands was fine.

She had watched me play several times so I knew she had an idea of what she was expected to do with the ball and therefore I gave her no specific directions or instructions. We both stood on the same side of the net—trying to hit over the net would have been foolish—and knowing that her hand-eye coordination was still minimal at that age, all I said was, "Try to hit the ball." She tried and missed almost every time but when she managed to hit it, she was delighted with her success. She liked the activity, she liked running after the ball, and she liked being out doing what she had seen Mommy and Daddy doing. The imposition of any rules would have been disastrous because she was not ready for them and they would have destroyed the sense of freedom she was experiencing.

I took great care to make the experience totally positive. As long as she was out there with me there was going to be no such thing as a failure for her. If she hit the ball it was great. If she missed, it was a terrific swing. If she ran after the ball, it was great running. There were no "nos." The specifics of the game didn't matter and when we finished she and I were both delighted to have played "tennis" together.

I knew that there would be plenty of time to add the rules and even then I could explain them one at a time as they became necessary. My daughter apparently enjoyed her outings with me because we continued to play together until she began to play with her own friends. At that point I stepped out of the picture.

Of course, I could have done just the opposite, as I saw a father doing not long ago. I watched as he told his five-year-old exactly how to hold a full-size tennis racket, how to stand and move when the ball approached, how to swing for a low shot and a high shot, the right form for the serve, and all the rest. The boy tried hard but the racket was too heavy and too long for him to handle and the father's instructions, though accurate, were too difficult to follow. I don't know what eventually happened, but it's my guess that what should have been a nice father and son experience turned into something less than pleasant, especially for the youngster.

The personal importance of winning and losing. When children are small, the concept of winning and losing doesn't exist. This couldn't be more healthy psychologically. When a child reaches the age of two, winning and losing are more like having or not having, that is, the terms have no greater meaning than sharing, which I mentioned above. When a child reaches age four, however, winning and losing become identifiable though they should still have little importance. In my experience, this is where parents enter the picture. I realize that in today's competitive world, winning is supposed to be important, but for a competitive parent to impose this concept full force on a child is a big mistake with big consequences. The following case illustrates the point.

About a year ago, a mother came to the office with her daughter because she was concerned with the girl's seemingly chronic state of depression. At that time, Katie was only seven and depression among seven-year-olds is unusual. I found her to be not only depressed, but full of anxieties, and I also found that those anxieties were more imagined than real. I quickly discovered the reason for her fears.

At age four, Katie's parents had enrolled her in a skating class with a professional teacher. The father, a nonathlete, had opposed the idea because he thought the girl was too young, but the mother, an active skater all her life, felt Katie would have potential and therefore, it was important to start her as early as possible.

There were twenty or so youngsters, all four and five, in the group and the coach worked them hard on the basics of figure skating in much the same way he would train adults. Every six weeks the class was tested on some aspect of what they had learned and those who passed earned merit badges and moved on to the next level; those who failed were held back. The sense of failure for those who did not pass had to be acute. Not only did their friends move ahead of them, but they were looked on by their peers and their parents in much the same way that a child who is held back in regular school is looked on—as a failure.

In conversations with the mother, I was told that Katie seemed to be progressing well with her skating but also that each week she protested vigorously about going to her class. Despite the child's protests about the rigors of the lessons and her worry about winning merit badges and getting promoted, the mother insisted that she continue in the school. The father continued to make objections, but since he was having no effect his protests were more pro forma than serious.

The real problem developed when, at age six, Katie started to fall a bit behind the girls who had entered the school with her. She had not been held back yet, but it seemed that she soon would be. The coach had a conference with Katie and her mother in which they had discussed the girl's slowing development and since that meeting Katie had been filled with anxiety, especially on Saturday mornings.

After a few sessions in my office it was clear to me that this little girl's fears and her depression were firmly grounded in her skating experiences because she seemed perfectly healthy in every other way. But the extent of her fear over the classes had virtually destroyed her appetite, was causing her to lose sleep, and she had even developed a skin rash which was also part of her psychological response to the pressure of her skating classes.

My first recommendation was that Katie be removed from the classes on a trial basis to see if some of her symptoms would be relieved. The father agreed readily and the mother reluctantly. Not surprisingly, three weeks later they called to tell me that their daughter was back to normal and they were going to put her back in the skating school.

I discussed this with Katie, who told me she was afraid to start again because she wasn't good enough to compete and she knew it. I've found that children have a keen sense of their own abilities and when a child reacts as Katie did, I am usually convinced. I advised the parents against further classes, at least at that time. I also suggested that they discuss this with Katie.

Fortunately, both parents were concerned enough about their child's overall mental health to do so, and smart enough to listen to what the child had to say. The lessons were dropped, the skating career was put on hold, and Katie started to eat and sleep normally again.

For Katie's mother, winning had been very important. It had not been very important for Katie. Fortunately, Katie had been able to make the judgment for herself and will approach future decisions of importance with a sense of herself and her ability to make those decisions.

This does not mean that winning isn't important or that the lessons learned in competition, the thrill of doing your best, the joy of success aren't all valid sensations. It only means that when the emphasis is placed solely on winning or advancing, as in the case of Katie, most of the healthy aspects of athletics are lost.

If there is one basic truism in sports, it's that winning isn't inevitable, but losing is. It's trite but true that only one person or one team wins. In baseball, where a .300 batting average is good hitting, seven out of ten times up the .300 hitter becomes a loser. Successful pitchers get knocked out of the game more often than they finish and even if they finish they can still be the loser. In tennis, almost as many shots go outside the line as inside. Even the best individuals and the best teams eventually lose, if not during this season then the next.

Children need very little preparation for winning—most take it in stride—but there are two important factors to keep in mind about winning. The first is that winning should be done graciously and that opponents should not be belittled. The second is that winning today doesn't mean winning tomorrow.

On the other side of the coin, however, it is important that parents prepare their children for the experience of losing, since losing is a potentially damaging emotional experience for a child. We don't usually prepare our children for failure, but we should. Here are some hints on how to do it.

You can begin by explaining some of the facts mentioned above about batting averages, tennis shots, etc. Also mention that losing is inevitable but that it is only an episode, a transient event in life not the whole of life. Explain that you can be on the losing side many times but that over a period of time, the wins and losses tend to balance out.

Tell the child that losing has absolutely nothing to do with self-worth, that an individual's personal value is not measured by

the number of hits he gets in a baseball season or the number
of perfectly skated figure-eights. Therefore, winning and losing
should have no effect whatever on self-esteem. You might also
mention that despite all the talk and promotional hype about
"winning" in life, particularly in the America of the 1980s, that
particular emphasis is simply not valid.

Once again, remember that you, as the parent, are the
trustee, the guardian of your child's emotional well-being, and it
is your responsibility to put these matters into perspective.

Acceptance and credibility among peers: Peer approval is
another important element in child development and it often
comes as a result of athletic participation and prowess, though
skill is less important than playing the game. In fact, there is no
quicker way for a child to win acceptance in a group than to
show he or she can play the game whatever that game may be.

A typical example of this dynamic can be found when a child
enters a new school. There is always a built-in reticence to
accept the new boy or girl in the class and a feeling of loneliness
and isolation is not uncommon among children when they are
first thrown into a new school situation.

All that is usually necessary to break the social ice, however,
is for the newcomer to perform adequately in a game whether
it's dodge ball, jump rope, or tag. A good showing almost guaran-
tees that the word will quickly spread around the class that "the
new kid is okay." After that, social acceptance is virtually
secured.

This acceptance is obviously good for the child's self-esteem
as well, because later he will receive further affirmation of his
worth through the approval of his peers, that is, being chosen to
be on the team, asked to meet the group after school, and invited
to come to the park on Saturday. Approval from a coach and
praise from parents is also important, but recognition from one's
peers, at any age, is a potent factor in the formation of a healthy
ego.

Studies done on the subject of peer acceptance and athletic
participation indicate that children who are separated from athletic and sports experiences, even just from participation in
recess at school, feel a distinct sense of separateness, a sense of
not being part of the group in any way. This is true even for the
most intellectually oriented youngster who is stereotypically
uninvolved in sports primarily because he wants to be. The
innermost feelings of those youngsters, as revealed in the

research, indicates a desire to be part of the group by playing games with the group.

It's true that this same youngster is often uninvolved because he feels a sense of inadequacy about his ability to play the game well. As a defense against failure when he does try to participate, he tells himself that sports are unimportant. Yet, the studies show the reality is different and that he would be very pleased to participate at any level. Athletics are such an integral part of our society that given the opportunity, virtually all children would choose to be involved in sports in some fashion or another. Inside everyone, apparently, is the interest or need to participate in the sporting life.

The opportunity for parents to give unqualified support to a child. Support is one of life's neglected skills. It costs nothing to give someone a pat on the back because you like them or to compliment them on a job well done, but it seems to be a tremendous price to pay for some people. Many times the price is even too high when it comes to supporting and approving the actions of our own children. I firmly believe we only make it through this world by supporting each other in one fashion or another, and the psychological impact of that support is profoundly positive. And it is the same whether it's a boss supporting an employee, a spouse supporting a spouse, or a parent supporting child.

It's possible that in the course of daily life there aren't enough opportunities for giving the kind of unqualified support that recognizes every effort as good and positive. I doubt that this is the case, but if it is, then athletics is absolutely unique in offering this opportunity in thousands of ways.

When it comes to supporting children, I call it the "apple of my eye" dynamic. The most important thing a parent can give a child is absolute approval, the recognition by the parent that whatever the child does is great. Athletics provides parents with the chance to do this in abundance.

The "apple of my eye" dynamic means simply that the parent gives unqualified, uncensored, absolute approval to the child for taking part in the activity whether it's throwing a ball or jumping in the swimming pool. There are many ego-building factors in childhood, but the most crucial is that the child have the experience of knowing he or she is the greatest, the most important thing in the parent's life. If I had to pick only one concept to pass on to parents it would be this message.

This is how it relates to athletics. Unlike other life situations, games themselves provide the perfect vehicle for parents to give their children a positive response. School doesn't offer the same opportunities because it is a more complex situation. In school, a certain amount of parental pressure—and anxiety—is normal because of the direct correlation between doing well in school and future success in life. It is obvious to parent, teacher, and student alike that they have a lot more at stake.

But despite the platitudes about the playing fields of Eton, doing well in sports does not correlate at all with doing well in life, with being brave, a good leader, or a good follower. So virtually every time a child plays any game, the parent is presented with a positive parenting opportunity. Each time a child touches a ball his father or mother can say, "Good catch," "Nice try," "Great," "That's terrific." It doesn't matter a bit whether the child is catching, trying hard, or doing anything terrific, the point is the parent can tell him that what he's doing is good and important.

In athletics, there is nothing the child can possibly do that a parent can't convert into a positive event. The idea is to reinforce participation and not to demean the child's efforts for any reason. Athletics provides even the most inept and uncoordinated child with the opportunity to receive parental approval.

So, if you can only give your child one special feeling, make it the feeling of thinking that he is the best thing that has ever happened to this planet. If you do nothing else as a parent, you will have given a tremendous gift. You will undoubtedly do other important things later on, but you shouldn't stop doing this even when your child becomes an adult.

$$\nabla \qquad \nabla \qquad \nabla$$

△ THE MAJOR STAGES OF A CHILD'S PHYSICAL DEVELOPMENT △

A child goes through three major stages of physical development: birth to age three, ages four to seven, and ages eight to eleven. Because of individual physical variations, these changes don't happen on a precise schedule, but the ranges are accurate for most children give or take a few months.

Stage One, birth to age three, is what I call the pre-athletic period. In these years the emphasis should be on physicality and movement in general, body-awareness and body control, and the pure exhilaration of physical activity. All activities should be informal, fun-oriented, spontaneous, frivolous, and light-hearted. Believe it or not, I've seen fathers coaching their sons on how to throw a baseball with accuracy at age two. This is not the kind of exposure I'm talking about.

In Stage Two, ages four to seven, children should be given their first informal opportunity to participate in what can be loosely defined as organized sports. These activities, kicking a ball around the yard, ice or roller skating at a local rink, are not structured and require no real instruction by parents or anyone else. This first exposure gives the child the chance to further develop his or her body awareness and coordination through sports activities.

At this point, rules are irrelevant unless a child asks about them. For example, if tennis is one of the activities that interest your child, the important elements are the sensation of hitting the ball and developing hand-eye coordination, not hitting it over the net or inside the lines. The same is true in other sports. In soccer, kicking the ball is the point, not putting it in a goal, and in baseball, catching and hitting the ball are the goals, not the foul lines or running the bases.

Children will pick up the rules as they play and as their interest develops, and this will come either from watching the game played on the field or on television or asking questions about specific points as they become important.

A child's coordination is far from fully developed at this stage, so sports that require catching or hitting a ball will be more difficult than those that require kicking a ball, riding a bicycle, roller and ice skating, swimming, or the martial arts. These latter activities, therefore, should be emphasized.

Remember, all sports require coordination for excellence, but not many require good coordination in order to participate at the basic level. The physical and emotional benefits are derived through participation not through excellent performance.

Coaching or any kind of serious instruction is still premature at age six and besides, there is no way, except in a few unusual cases, that it can have a positive long-term benefit. There is no proof that early coaching will make a child a champion, though there are many coaches who claim this is the case. A child who starts early may have a brief advantage in sports but not in life. It is the same when a child reads at age four and his friend doesn't read until age six. When they are both eight, there will be little difference, if any, in their abilities. Parents need to be patient.

In Stage Three, ages eight to eleven, a child's coordination is sufficient to start playing sports that require more complex and difficult athletic skills. It is at this point that the talented youngster and his parents should begin to think about some form of coaching if the goal of the youngster is to eventually compete at the college and possibly at the professional levels in his or her chosen sport.

The next three chapters will examine these three stages in more detail.

4

The Movement Years— Zero to Three

I URGE ALL parents to give their children an athletic experience as early as possible, regardless of whether the parents themselves have any real interest in athletics and sports or not. Physical activity is such a vital factor in early childhood development that I don't think it can begin too early.

But even as I encourage you to provide this opportunity I also implore you to make these first experiences (and later ones as well) as much fun as possible. To do otherwise is to risk long-term psychological damage to your child and strained family relations that can last a lifetime. This may sound severe, but my clinical experience has demonstrated the truth of that statement.

This chapter is about three things: (1) the types of activities that are appropriate for young children; (2) when to start these activities; and (3) making it fun.

One thing I find very discouraging when I talk with parents, coaches, and athletes (even young athletes), is that the word missing from their sports vocabularies is that most basic of all childhood concepts, "fun." I say this is discouraging, and I'm speaking here not only as a psychologist but as a parent and a sports fan, because, until a youngster reaches the age of eleven or twelve, sports are really play and nothing more. And play should be fun. In fact, what is play if it isn't fun?

Interestingly, this concept does not change with age. Even after childhood, sports should still be fun, even for those athletes with professional aspirations and those athletes who are professionals. Unfortunately, I know from talking with the athletes in my practice that this is not often the case.

Take the example of Bjorn Borg, the phenomenal Swedish tennis star who was the best player in the world for several years. Borg gained international fame and earned a considerable financial fortune with his tennis game, yet he retired from active competition in his mid-20s, the prime of his tennis-playing days. Among the reasons that he gave at the time was the fact that the game wasn't fun anymore. Tennis is a perfect example here because the nature of the game is such that players begin to compete for money at a very young age.

Yet the same thing happens to a lesser degree in almost every sport. The difference is we don't hear anything about it when a high school or college star in basketball, swimming, or whatever decides to call it quits because the game isn't fun anymore. Not all of these athletes would say that their reason for quitting was that the fun had gone out of the game, but many would say that it was part of the reason for their decision.

A young person whose sports activities don't leave time for anything outside that activity—for socializing, for family, for school work, for doing nothing at all—can suffer from more than burn-out. The constant pressure to succeed, whether applied by a parent, by a coach, by the public, or by the athlete himself, can be crippling to the young psyche.

Not long ago, a father, a former professional football player, came to me for guidance. Jack told me he had come from a sports-minded and highly competitive family in which all five brothers and three sisters had become top-flight athletes at the college level. One of his brothers had gone on to a professional career in baseball, another had become a college football coach, one sister was a champion cyclist. Jack himself had had a successful college football career and gone on to the pros. He played very well in his rookie season but was injured in his second year and never fully recovered from knee surgery. At age twenty-four he was forced to retire.

He went to work as an insurance salesman and married when he was thirty. He and his wife had one son and one daughter. He said his life after sports had not been a smashing success, at least not in light of his life as an athlete. After a few years he tired of the insurance business and decided to devote as much time as possible to turning his son into a football player. He pursued that course with determination, and though he didn't view his work with his son as an experiment in creating an athletic machine, he acknowledged that it certainly could be construed that way.

Now he had a problem and needed help. The problem, Jack told me, revolved around his son, who was a talented fifteen-year-old athlete who competed, and starred in, high school baseball, football and basketball. Jack had already had feelers from several college recruiters who had seen his son Tommy in action and he sensed that he had a winner in his son. But now, at the apex of his high school career, it seemed Tommy was losing his interest in competition. Jack was trying to convince him that this was the time when it was important to "pour it on" not slack off, but he was not having much luck.

As the father talked, I began to understand why Tommy was backing away from sports. Jack said he had always wanted a boy and when Tommy was born, he took a football to the hospital and asked the nurse to put it in the boy's crib. There was always a ball of some sort in the boy's bed and when he was able to sit up and move around, his father made sure that there was always a ball nearby. When Tommy was able to grasp objects his father put a ball in his hand and helped him squeeze it and roll it from hand to hand. As Tommy grew, the father focused more and more attention on the boy, actually quitting his job in order to spend more time at the task of molding a champion.

When Tommy was only eighteen months old, Jack began taking him to sports events and when they watched television together they always watched sports instead of cartoons or other children's programs. "I kept at it," Jack told me, "because Tommy always loved sports even when he was small. For God's sake, his first word was 'ball'."

It's certainly not surprising that Tommy showed a "spontaneous" interest in sports as soon as he was able to speak. That interest had been carefully nurtured by the father. Many years before it was appropriate, Jack started priming Tommy for a career in sports. He even put Tommy's name on the list for the Pop Warner football program and Little League at age three, even though it was premature and unnecessary to do so.

Through a combination of genes, parental coaching, and parental pressure to perform, Tommy developed into a truly special athlete. At age six, he was the envy of the boys in his neighborhood and Jack, as well as Tommy, became the object of the attention and adulation of other parents. Even at that age Tommy was able to throw a football twenty yards and hit a baseball hard and long. The adoration of his father and his peers raised Tommy's level of self-esteem to the point where he actually thought he was a special person, set apart from the rest of the children his age because of his athletic skills. This level of self-esteem, so valuable normally, soon turned to cockiness and bravado, which was only natural under these circumstances.

Tommy's mother, also an athletic person, was not as pleased as his father about the amount of time and effort being spent on Tommy's development as an athlete. Jack told me he had some discussions and some serious arguments with his wife about it, but that he had prevailed and she had said little about the issue in the last three years. He said, however, that he felt she was harboring a lot of resentment against him and that some of that resentment was spilling over onto Tommy and causing Tommy to turn against sports and him. Jack's recognition of the problems was fine, but his concern wasn't so much that these problems were cropping up, but that they "could effect Tommy's performance."

About a year ago, Jack said, Tommy began rebelling against the daily routine of playing whatever sport was in season. He said he knew he was good and that was all that was necessary for him to know. He felt he had proved himself to his father and didn't owe him anything. The boy became much less cocky and seemed to be satisfied with what he had accomplished, at peace with himself. He had also begun to develop an interest in girls and was suddenly happier spending his time with one or two special girl friends than snapping towels with the boys in the locker room.

Jack told me that he and the boy had a dozen verbal fights about the boy's change of heart and that one afternoon Tommy had said: "It's too much work to keep playing. I want to have some fun." This comment infuriated Jack and he hit his son. The boy fought back and the two had not spoken since. It was after the fist fight that Jack had come to see me.

Frankly, you don't have to be a psychologist to have a general understanding of what happened in this family and what caused it. Jack himself was the problem, not Tommy. The foundation for Jack's problems was twofold: his upbringing in a highly competitive family, and the knee injury that had prevented him from proving himself on the football field. Jack was living vicariously through his son, who was fulfilling the father's unfulfilled personal expectations. Given his family background, Jack could have pushed Tommy to a sports career anyway, but the career-ending injury was the pivotal element in the combination of forces acting on Jack.

This resulted in Jack's compulsive need to drive Tommy, who initially responded positively because he was too young to know any different. Later he followed his father's guidance because he wanted to please him, but ultimately, as he matured, he rebelled against his father's continual autocratic insistence and control.

Fortunately, Tommy had a strong enough ego to resist his father's fanatic influence. The average young man might not have been as strong, might have had more fear of his father's rejection and continued to play despite his own feelings. I suspect that his mother's support, however tentative, had something to do with his strength in the face of his father's insistence.

The whole episode created a rift between father and son and between husband and wife which battered the entire family structure. Athletics are usually a unifying family experience, but in this case, and in cases where pressure takes away the fun, they can be unpleasant and divisive. This strips away all the positives that athletics can offer.

In my work I've noted one thing that is common to all children: the desire to have fun. The prospect of having fun, of enjoying something, is what draws children to play a game, read a book, listen to music, or paint a picture. If the athletic experience (or reading or listening to music or painting) is not fun, it can be painful and cause anxiety even in very young children. Overzealous parents pushing for their child to "achieve" should take note that a child will acquiesce to your wishes initially but as soon as the experience produces anxiety and fear the child will shy away and may avoid the activity, as well as the parent, permanently.

Jack's story illustrates the need for vigilance on the part of parents, a vigilance that you can test for yourself. The logic of what I'm saying is clear, but I realize that the practice is difficult because the progression can be so subtle as to be unrecognizable. But the fact is, enthusiasm can lead to obsessiveness.

This is something you should consider even in the movement years. So even if you don't feel you are pushing your child and that there is no way you can be taking the fun out of something that should be enjoyable, ask yourself the following questions:

1. Is the idea in the back of my mind that my child should, if he shows the talent I expect, eventually receive professional instruction?

2. Do I find myself fantasizing about my child playing pro sports?

3. Do I strongly urge my child to watch sports on television?

4. Are trips to the stadium a ritual like going to church?

5. Do I enjoy bragging about my child's athletic accomplishments?

6. Do I take time off from work to help my child in his physical development?

7. Do I and my spouse agree on the question of our child's involvement in sports?

8. Does my child resist my suggestions to play, practice, or become more involved?

In light of the case history of Jack and Tommy, you will be able to evaluate your own answers to these questions. And as you can see from the case history, these questions are not premature.

Pay particular attention to question eight, since it is perhaps the most important of all. Even little children know what they like when it comes to food and they also know what they like when it comes to athletic or movement activity. If there is resistance, either verbal or physical, you are well advised to slow down and back off. There may be any number of reasons for your child's reactions—including the fact that whatever it is that he is doing may be physically painful—but even when this doesn't seem to be the case, heed the warning signals and back off. There is plenty of time.

Though this case history clearly points out the dangers inherent in applying too much pressure in sports, it is equally applicable to the parent who applies pressure on a child to become a doctor, lawyer, accountant, insurance salesman, or even an excellent student.

The story of Jack and Tommy is an example of the most severe form of overt pressure put on a child by a parent obsessed with his own feelings of inadequacy and attempting to live his unfulfilled dreams through the exploits of his child.

There are less overt, much more subtle types of pressure which I want to mention briefly. Parents are teachers, but we often find ourselves instructing where no instruction is necessary. I suspect it's part of the "don't" syndrome, but it is less automatic because it requires some followup. The phrases to watch for include:

▷ You're not doing that right.

▷ Let me show you how to do that.

▷ Try to do it right the first time.

▷ Stop doing that until you can do it right.

▷ It's time you learned how to do this yourself.

▷ I've showed you this ten times. Why can't you get it?

▷ You'll never learn.

▷ I'll do it for you.

Make no mistake, you are the child's primary teacher, and you are entitled to use any approach you see fit. These particular phrases are pointed out not because they are harmful in themselves when used occasionally, but when they become part of the daily vocabulary the parent uses with the child, and they are said in a tone of voice that tells a child he or she is incapable, their use can be damaging. Eventually the constant badgering can cause a deep rift between parent and child.

Let me point out once more that the psyches of young children are sensitive and fragile. The things adults say and take for granted are often interpreted negatively by a child. Certainly, *no* and *don't* are words that must be used from time to time, but when they are overused they are destructive to a child's self-esteem and confidence.

Possibly the worst example of early instruction I've ever seen was in observing a father teaching his two-year-old son the basics of running. Two-year-olds walk and run naturally. Since their ability to control their gross motor movements is not fully developed, they don't run in a coordinated way regardless of the amount of instruction heaped on them. Yet I saw this father explaining the fine points of running to his son in the manner of a coach. He told the boy to get up on his toes, be sure to swing his arms, keep his head up, his eyes straight ahead, and to breathe through his mouth. Of course, the boy was unable to do these things and the father was getting more and more frustrated in his efforts. The child was finally reduced to tears and the father was flabbergasted at the boy's inability to perform one of the "simplest" of physical movements.

I don't know if the child protested to his father, but be aware that just as there are phrases to watch for in your communication with your child, there are telltale phrases to listen for in your child's speech at times when you are trying to give instructions. Some of these are:

▷ That's too hard.

▷ I'm tired.

▷ Let's do it tomorrow.

▷ I don't want to.

▷ I can't.

▷ I want to do something else.

▷ I'm not going to.

▷ Let's stop now.

▷ This is no fun.

▷ I'm thirsty.

These are not casual remarks. When your child says these and similar things, he is really telling you that he is not happy with what is going on and would rather do something else. This doesn't mean that the activity can't be tried another time. What it does mean is that the child doesn't consider the activity within his capabilities at the moment, and knowing this, he or she is reluctant to continue, even fearful of doing so. These warnings from the child are valid, they contain a message, so don't force the issue. Simply put the activity aside and try it again in a month or six months or even a year. Remember that fun is the key. If it is not fun for the child it won't be fun for you either.

△ What Parents Should Do to Encourage Zero- to Three-Year-Olds △

Given these "go slow" signals, what kinds of movements are appropriate for the zero- to three-year-old child?

When I use the word movement, I'm really talking about just that. From the first day, babies kick, they wave their arms, they squeeze their hands, they move their heads, and they toss from side to side. A baby will continue to move like this for two to three months in the crib and then begin to roll over. This rolling continues until the leg and arm muscles are strong enough to support the body. Crawling is the next step, and then the child begins to stand while holding on for support. By eleven or twelve months, most children are walking and beginning to climb.

Now you can begin to introduce your child to his physical being by letting him experiment and become comfortable with his body and learn to enjoy the visceral pleasure that comes from physical activity.

No instructions are necessary. Just provide an atmosphere that encourages natural movement and create opportunities for that movement. Confine your child as little as possible. Physically and psychologically I'm opposed to playpens because they are designed for control. An area only four feet by four feet is restrictive and drastically limits movement. Playpens, in fact, are for parents—that is, they allow the parent to move freely without worrying about the location of the child.

It is a sounder practice to "baby-proof" the house in the main area where the baby is going to be. Remove dangerous objects, cover electrical outlets, and put up gates and latches where necessary. This essentially creates a large play area or playpen, if you will, but it's big enough for the child to really move around.

A large open area encourages movement, encourages a child to crawl, roll, to begin to develop dexterity. When crawling, as much room as possible is desirable, and when the baby begins to walk and climb, a large area is much more hospitable.

Keep soft, child-size balls of various sizes and textures around for pushing and rolling. Introduce soft toys and puzzles into the environment because they provide opportunities to develop manual dexterity. Mobiles are also valuable because they help develop coordinated eye movements. Together, these things encourage movement, physicality, comfort with the body, a sense of space and a certain command of that space.

Outside play, in the yard or the park, is the logical next step. Swings, jungle gyms, slides, and ladders are safe when there is a parent to supervise the activity and climbing and swinging add to the child's sense of mobility and knowledge about spatial relations.

This acquiring of knowledge by the baby all takes place sub-consciously, of course. The child isn't saying to itself, "Now I'm moving my arms and I feel good about doing it and I can sense that there is space around me and I know how I fit in that space." But that is what is happening in the baby's head and it is the reason for movement activities.

When the time is right, scooters, tricycles, and small bicycles with training wheels, roller skates with plastic wheels, and ice skates with double runners should be added to the environment and more and more time should be spent in larger spaces. Throwing balls improves coordination and stretches muscles, and kicking the ball, which takes less coordination than throwing, should be encouraged. But note that even at age two and three it is still too early for a child to catch a ball. In fact, any time a child catches a ball at this age it is pure luck, since hand-eye coordination is still underdeveloped.

The movement goals in this time period are simply to allow and encourage the child to use his body, to be physical, mobile, and active, and to begin to develop his or her reflexes. There is nothing more to it.

For the parent, know yourself, be aware that this is where the obsession with performance begins, slow up, let your child's skills develop naturally.

Involving Fathers

There is one other point I want to make in this chapter: This kind of movement activity provides opportunities for fathers, specifically fathers, to have experiences with their children. This is important for two reasons:

1. Recent studies indicate that the importance of the father in the developmental process is considerably greater than psychologists thought in the past.

2. Athletics is one of the socially accepted ways for a father to be close, physical, and involved with his child—boy or girl.

Until a few years ago, psychologists felt the mother was by far the dominant figure in a child's life. After all, in most families, the mother is the primary nurturer, companion, guide, teacher, friend, and disciplinarian of the child. That thinking is changing in light of recent findings about the importance of the father at all stages of a child's development. That's where athletics comes into the picture.

There are few enough opportunities for a father to get close to his child and athletics is one that serves the purpose exceptionally well. Playing together, in even the most casual way, means being with the child in a nonthreatening situation.

These research findings also uncovered information that bears directly on the incidence of homosexuality in males. The conventional view has been that homosexuality in boys was primarily the result of a problem or problems the child experiences with the mother. Now, it appears that in more than 50 percent of the cases studied, male homosexuality was more likely attributable to the absence of a relationship with the father than it was to an overinvolvement on the part of the mother.

Again, sports offers an opportunity for fathers and sons to be together in a healthy, affectionate, warm, physical kind of way, a way that is eminently socially acceptable. The findings go on to say that the more contact a father has with a male child the less likely that child is to be homosexual as an adolescent or an adult.

CHAPTER

5

△ _____ △

The Sports Years— Four to Seven

B E AWARE THAT human development is not an exact science. The benchmarks for physical and emotional changes, especially in children, vary from child to child. Some children begin walking as early as nine months while others don't walk until they are eighteen months old or even older. Teeth come in at different speeds and speech develops early in some children and considerably later in others. These variations are no cause for concern, though I've heard parents bragging about the number of teeth their child has as if it was some special accomplishment that was due to the parents' superior genes.

After the age of two, physical size varies enormously and by the age of five the differences make one youngster appear to be at least seven while another may look more like he's three. For example, the normal range in height and weight of five-year-olds may vary by as much as six inches and thirty pounds and there is no reason to worry if your child falls at either end of this scale.

The range of emotional and intellectual maturity is just as great. One four-year-old may be completely comfortable in social

△

situations with children and adults and another may not have any concept of socialization; one may read and write by the age of three and another may not do either. Again, there is no cause for alarm in either case.

Physical coordination develops at highly variable rates in children, particularly in the early years. One three-year-old may run in a very coordinated way and another may stumble over his shadow. Coordination also tends to fluctuate in youngsters. That is, on Monday a given-four-year old may be able to hit and catch a ball with some skill and on Wednesday the same child may not be able to perform the task at all.

So, though I've created a division between ages three and four in the development of a child's athletic activities, there really is no clear-cut dividing line that says a child of three is not ready for certain physical activities and a child of four is ready. Parents are the best judges of a child's progress, so each parent will have to determine what stage his child is in, what activities seem appropriate, without being a slave to chronological age.

The case of a five-year-old named Carol illustrates this point rather clearly. Carol, the daughter of a friend, showed remarkable coordination at the age of eighteen months. She was able to swim before she could walk and when she started to walk at eleven months, her father decided to try her on ice skates. At first he put her on double runners but within weeks he had her on single-blade skates. When they went skating, Carol was the talk of the rink. Then, suddenly, at about twenty-four months, virtually all of her coordination disappeared. Her parents were surprised and disturbed by this development, but when they asked me about it I assured them that this sort of thing happens frequently. About six months later, Carol started to regain her coordination and she has been developing at a normal rate ever since.

But regardless of emotional, intellectual, or physical maturity, a child who has been exposed to, and taken part in, movement activities in his first three years, will likely be more coordinated and show more interest in physical activity than a child who has been given limited opportunities or no opportunities at all to experience the joys of movement. Research also shows that the active child may very well be healthier as well, suffering from fewer colds and other minor childhood ailments.

Until about age four, even the physically active child plays games and watches games with little regard to the form of those games, and who wins and who loses has no importance. At this age, when a child watches games on television, the names of the teams and the players are pretty much of a blur, and all but the simplest rules are too abstract to comprehend. This is true whether the child is actually playing the game or watching the movement on the TV screen; action is the attraction because it is stimulating and exciting. This is why children run whenever they can; it is more exciting than walking.

At about age four, the physically active child who regularly plays games and watches games will quite naturally begin to ask his parents more pointed questions about sports and specific games. He or she will want to know "why" something is done the way it is done and not some other way, "how" to go about doing it, "what" the rules are and then "why" those rules say this or that.

Earlier, I talked about playing tennis with my four-year-old daughter. That example is apt once again. In the beginning stages of learning any sport a child can only be exposed to the absolute rudiments of the game. In tennis the minimum require-ment is that of holding the racket, swinging it, and trying to hit the ball. Nets, boundary lines, scores, and the other elements that make tennis distinctive are immaterial and bothersome at best and distracting and destructive at worst. In fact, the intro-duction of any of these "technical" elements will probably ruin any chance of enjoyment or achievement by the child for some time.

This is simply because the mechanics of the sport take so much energy and concentration that the child has to focus all of his or her attention on swinging the racket and trying to hit the ball. When the child hits it, the achievement is complete and clear and that is sufficient reward. It doesn't matter in the slight-est where the ball goes. With enough swings and enough hits, the child's confidence slowly increases and he or she can think about hitting the ball harder, farther, and straighter.

My daughter and I played our little game of hitting the ball back and forth by the side of the court for at least six months. I have to admit that I was getting anxious to explain some of the rules of the game, but I resisted the urge. Then one day she asked me some direct questions about the reason for the lines on the court and what the net was there for, and we were on the way. The important thing is that the interest in these facts came from her, not from me. The progression had been easy and natural.

So by the age four or five, the active child will be fairly familiar with his body and will have developed a sense of his own
physical capabilities and his own interests. Not only that, he will
have played often enough with his father or mother or other children and he will have watched enough events on television that
he will know the basics of some games.

△ What Parents Can Do To Encourage Four- to Seven-Year-Olds △

At this stage, based on the groundwork laid by you, it is safe to
begin offering your child choices in the world of more organized
activities. Keep in mind, however, that a four-year-old (even a
five- or six-year-old) is still a small child and encouragement
rather than direction or formalized coaching is necessary to
ensure his or her continued interest in sports. Parental pressure
to play will not work for long.

If you have made the effort to expose your child to a variety
of physical activities, your next step is to watch him over a period
of months to determine what sport or sports he seems to like
best. Don't press too hard to make this determination, however,
because some children like every sport and if that's the case
there is no need to focus on one at the expense of another. I don't
want you to get the impression that any decisions whatever need
to be made at this time. You'll only be looking for a general show
of interest on the part of your child.

And try not to be deceived or deceive yourself in this process.
Many childhood interests are formed by watching television, but
there may or may not be a connection between the sports your
child likes to watch on TV and those he likes to play. Some
youngsters like to watch football because of the action, the noise,
and the color, but when it comes to playing they would prefer to
play catch with a baseball rather than a football.

Here are some indicators you can look for. Does your child
seem to like:

▷ Individual sports like tennis and running

▷ Team sports like baseball and football

▷ Contact sports, like boxing and hockey

▷ Non-contact sports, like golf and racketball

▷ Sports with balls

▷ Sports without balls, like swimming and skiing

▷ Sports with equipment and uniforms

▷ Sports that require parental supervision

▷ Sports that don't need any supervision

If for some reason you can't tell much about your child's major interests simply by observing, then ask a few questions based on these indicators. Your questions should be casual, occasional, and should pose no threat whatever to the child's interests. Those questions might be something like the following:

▷ I've seen you playing basketball with Tommy. Is it fun? Is it more fun than football? Is it more fun than anything?

▷ Boy, the Super Bowl was exciting wasn't it? Would you like to play football some day?

▷ I think golf is kind of boring. What do you think?

▷ The Astros uniforms are great, aren't they?

▷ The great thing about running is you can do it all by yourself. Do you like to play by yourself more than with other people?

▷ Did you see the way the coach was talking to his players? I think that's a big help. What do you think?

▷ Did you see the way the coach was yelling at his players? What do you think about the way he treats them?

These questions are only suggestive, and there are obviously many others you can think of. Just make sure you take your cues from your child; don't make choices for him, don't feed him the answers you want, and remember that it isn't necessary to make any kind of firm choice among activities. You're only trying to gauge your child's interest.

Your attitude will obviously have an influence on your child's choice of athletic activities. In most cases, parents will begin by

exposing their child to their own favorite sports, and this is fine
as long as the child's interest lies in that direction.

In those cases where the parent is not sports-minded in any
way, the child's decision will be based entirely on his or her own
feelings and those feelings should be recognized and supported.

How do you lend that support? Whether you're a sports
addict or not, there are certain things you can do that are neither
intrusive or gratuitous.

1. If equipment is necessary, you can buy what's needed. Be
sure to buy child-size baseball gloves, tennis rackets, etc., since
they are more comfortable for small hands and the undeveloped
musculature of a child. Don't buy the most expensive models of
any piece of equipment because your child will soon outgrow
them.

2. Play the sport of his choice with your child, and if for some
reason you can't, try to find a friend who is willing to play with
your child.

3. Watch the sport on television or find games in your area
to watch live and talk about what you see in the games.

4. Talk about the sport as much as your child wants to talk.

5. Buy illustrated reading material about the sport that you
can share with your child.

6. Help your child set up a timetable with short- and long-
term goals regarding his favorite sport or sports. For example,
you may want to talk about the possibility of a summer sports
camp two or three years down the road.

All that said, try not to go overboard in your support. Temper
your enthusiasm with a wait-and-see attitude. That is, don't
make promises about the future that you aren't likely to keep.
And don't invest too much emotionally or financially, because a
child's interests change frequently and quickly. If you rush out
and buy the latest innovation in tennis rackets, you may find
yourself owning a piece of $150 equipment that won't help you
a bit with your golf game.

At the same time you're supporting your child in his or her
chosen sport of the moment, encourage the youngster to take up
more than one sport. Time spent in two or three seasonal sports

will give him or her a chance to experiment and will prevent the focus on one sport from becoming too intense. If necessary, you can use the argument that many good athletes play several sports and some even manage professional careers in two sports.

△ COACHING AND PROFESSIONAL TRAINING △

There is a school of thought that says a talented child must begin to receive professional coaching at a very young age in order to achieve success in any sport. Internationally known coaches in gymnastics, figure skating, and ballet loudly claim that it's absolutely necessary for a child to begin serious professional training for these athletic activities by age six or seven at the latest. I'll concede that it *may* be important for a child's muscles to be trained early in order to perform movements perfectly when the youngster reaches the age of competition or performance at twelve or thirteen.

But the claim that such early training is necessary for success has no real basis in fact. It's true that young children are trainable and that those who get training early have a head start, but a child who starts later, with more physical and emotional maturity, quickly closes any training gap. It's my contention that professional coaching, or even serious amateur coaching from parents or friends, is not only premature at age six or seven but doesn't produce the desired results in the end. That is, *concentrated early training doesn't produce a better athlete.*

But more importantly, even if early training did produce a superstar by age ten, it wouldn't be worth the psychological cost to the child and the family. That doesn't mean that parents who think their child has the interest and the potential to be a good athlete should not begin to think of focusing that child's attention on a specific sport or at least narrowing down the child's interest to two or three areas. This can be done by observation and judicious questioning, but the point remains that coaching for a child in this age group is inappropriate and potentially harmful.

From a physical point of view, and perhaps more importantly from an emotional point of view, the pressure of the rigorous dis-

cipline of coaching or training can be very damaging to a youngster. Thus, in my opinion the conventional coaching wisdom is
not only unproven by also unwise. The following case history will
give you an example of what I mean.

One of America's most promising young female gymnasts, a
good candidate for the U.S. Olympic team, follows a training routine that is not only damaging her physically but has completely
taken away her childhood and her life as a teenager. She is now
seventeen; she began her rigorous training at the age of twelve.

First, let's take a look at the physical cost of that training. For
the last five years she has been training five hours a day, five
days a week, fifty-two weeks a year. She maintains her 5' 1", 104-
pound body on a diet of 800 calories a day, even though her exercises alone demand a richer caloric intake than that. She admits,
"Sometimes I don't know where I get the energy to train." No
wonder.

Our Olympic hopeful begins each training session with a
warmup routine that she says "feels as painful as it looks." During her sessions she practices the four Olympic events—vault,
balance beam, uneven parallel bars, and floor exercises—and
follows that with a half hour of strength training.

"I never go through a day without feeling stiff," she says, "and
I don't mean muscle soreness." In 1985, she broke her leg in a
fall but she managed to recover and perform again even though
she "wasn't too sure she could come back." Of this and the rest
of her training, she says, "I guess my joints will hurt for the rest
of my life."

Since she was a preteenager, this young lady has been depriv-
ing her body nutritionally at the same time she has been tor-
menting it physically. She has been severely injured and she
realizes that she will have to live with pain the rest of her life.
She doesn't yet know that the pain will become even more severe
when her joints develop arthritis, which they will. This is a high
price to pay for a crack at an Olympic medal.

The emotional picture is just as grim. Though I don't know
the young lady personally, I do know that in situations like this
the child is continually pressured to perform by parents, coaches,
and peers. This takes a terrible emotional toll because it forces
the child to feel guilty whenever she performs at a level lower
than that expected by her various mentors and her competition.
At the same time, she has been deprived of what could be called
a normal social life since her school day is arranged around her

workout schedule, all her friends are gymnasts, and she is not allowed to keep the hours that a normal teenager would keep. In short, she has missed virtually all the pleasures of growing up including the opportunity to have a variety of friends, to enjoy food, and to have the freedom to spend her time as she wishes. Yes, she has met other youngsters in the narrow world of gymnastics, she has had the privilege of working with top coaches, and she has traveled widely, but in my opinion the cost is too high.

I'm quite sure visions of gold medals were dangled before this young athlete's eyes and that she was told she could be a champion when she began her training. But a twelve-year-old child is not intellectually capable of committing herself to this kind of life. In fact, in my experience, no child would make such a decision of her own free will so I have to conclude that it was a decision that was imposed on the girl by parents and coaches who are also the ones applying pressure for her to continue and achieve the goal they've established for her.

As I've said before, parents are responsible for their children. This case shows how parents can abdicate that responsibility and the results, in my mind, are very close to child abuse. Obviously, the same thing can happen when parents pressure their children to become musicians, doctors, or accountants, but the pressure to perform in these fields, though it may be destructive psychologically, is not destructive physically as well.

There will be more on this subject in Chapters 6 and 7.

6

△   △

Take the Pressure Off —
Ages Seven to Eleven

CHILDREN IN THE seven to eleven age range are neither fish nor fowl, as we used to say. Mentally, they are often mature enough to make some important decisions on their own about basic things, and most are able to control their emotions in normal social and private situations. Physically, the majority of children in this age range have enough motor control to be capable of performing the tasks required in daily life as well as those required by any sport.

Yet the range of variation—both physically and emotionally—in this five-year time span is probably greater than at any other period during a youth's development, even greater than those differences noted in the previous chapters.

Certainly, most seven-year-olds don't have the size or coordination to compete with eleven-year-olds, but I've seen some exceptional late-seven-year-olds who could. I've also seen ten-year-old boys who were big enough to play high school football and I've seen other ten-year-olds who were so small and frail they barely looked like they were ready for first grade. I've seen nine-

△

and ten-year-old-girls who were considerably bigger than most of the boys in their age group and I've seen others who were still small and full of baby fat. In fact, this is the age range in which many girls catch up with and surpass boys in size, coordination, and emotional maturity.

Size is a critical factor in sports performance at any age, of course, but a smallish boy or girl with good coordination can play rings around a larger child who is less coordinated, especially during this stage of development. Emotional maturity is less visible and consequently less definable. And it has little to do with size, although some very large and very small children have more difficulty socially and emotionally because they often become objects of the curiosity and finger pointing of other children.

What is less evident than size, coordination, and emotional development is the fact that the abilities of growing youngsters change rapidly until they reach the age of twelve or thirteen. So, a child who appears to have exceptional talent at age eight, a child who has to play with older boys and girls in order to play up to his or her capabilities, may not continue to develop that talent and may actually suffer an erosion of his or her skills as the body goes through its natural hormonal changes. Therefore, early judgments about talent are extremely difficult to make and should not be made until a child begins the maturing process that takes place at puberty.

The following case history will give you an idea of what can happen in this volatile transition period between childhood and adolescence. Not long ago, a father came to me for some advice. The man, a former big league baseball player, was concerned about his son Ron's lack of progress in Little League baseball and his concern was based on the fact that the boy appeared to have the makings of a genuine prodigy at age nine, and now, at twelve, he was playing less well than he ever had with the result that most of the other boys on the team were passing him by.

The father's concern was partly based on his own need for his son to excel, but it was also based on his son's personal desires to follow in his father's footsteps. This was not so much a case of parental pressure as a shared feeling between father and son that playing professional baseball was something worth pursuing.

Parents are not usually the best judges of a child's talent, even those parents who have played or coached the sport their child is playing. When this father told me his son displayed exceptional ability as early as age seven, I questioned his appraisal. Without seeing the child myself, the father's comments indicated to me that the boy did indeed have talent and even discounting the father's justifiable pride in his son, it seemed he had a case.

Since Ron had been old enough to grasp a ball, he had been prompted and encouraged by the father (and his mother, to a certain extent) to develop the skills he possessed. When he was only five he was sent to a two-week camp that specialized in baseball. According to the report from the camp director, the boy had shown outstanding ability and coordination for a child so young.

The following summer Ron went to a four-week camp and got rave notices from his coaches and he was being tabbed, even at that young age, as a potential professional prospect.

These various camps, the boy's equipment, the transportation and other attention he received from the family all cost money, and it was money the family really didn't have. In fact, the father, now the owner of a small tire business, took out a second mortgage on the family home in order to meet some of these expenses.

The problem was not that the father was having trouble facing the reality of the situation because, surprisingly, he was able to do so. Nor was his problem that he couldn't approach his son on the issues involved, because he could and did. The problem was that he wasn't able to convince his wife that there was a significant question about their son's level of real talent.

The primary point of contention from the mother's point of view was the fact that the family had invested all this money and time and emotion in the son's training and that money now looked like it had been "wasted." The wife wanted to place blame, and she was distributing it evenly between her husband and her son, and both were feeling guilty about their roles in what the mother called "a great deception."

I explained to the father that this was not an uncommon situation, that young prodigies in sports and other fields often reach a plateau in the immediate preteen years where their skills remain the same and those of the other players catch up. I pointed out to him that no one was at fault and no one was to blame. He told me that the family had gone into this with open eyes and that only reaffirmed my opinion that there was no blame to be assessed and certainly none should fall on the shoulders of the young boy, whose disappointment was going to be great enough. Finally, I tried to explain to him that the money hadn't been wasted at all and that in the long term, the entire family would come to realize that fact.

Several months later the father came to visit me one more time. He told me that he had finally gotten a positive response from his wife and that after many hours of discussion she had admitted that her disappointment was in the destruction of her fantasy of having a professional athlete for a son, someone she could brag about to the neighbors and go see at the ball park, and that this had been a much greater problem than the monetary outlay. I felt they were on the right track and though I have not heard from them since, I have the feeling that things turned out satisfactorily.

This case history illustrates the principal danger in the early assessment of physical talent, even when that assessment is made by someone qualified to do it. The danger is in assuming that athletic skill and coordination continue to improve as the young body matures. Some youngsters are very fast starters and reach the peak of their skills before puberty. These children stand out sufficiently from the crowd to be considered prodigies in their preteen years. Others start more slowly, but when their skills begin to develop, they come on with such a rush that they pass their peers as if the others were standing still.

There is no way to predict this situation, and that's one of the reasons I advise parents to put off all serious coaching until their child is eleven or twelve. At that time, most of the changes in a child's body will have occurred and more considered judgments can be made about that child's potential.

△ THE REQUIREMENTS OF A LIFE IN SPORTS CAN BE DESTRUCTIVE △

One other point I want to make here: A life in sports is not normal. There is nothing normal about exceptional athletic performance, or the rigors of physical and mental training, or the adulation of peers and total strangers. It is not an easy life, though it can be tremendously stimulating to the ego and financially rewarding in the bargain. The physical strains and pressures of top sports performance, and the mental strains and pressures on top performers, are difficult for virtually every athlete to handle. Therefore, our baseball player who was not as talented as first thought and had to change his course in midstream was lucky to discover the fact at age eleven instead of age eighteen. It was actually a blessing in disguise for him and his family. He and his mother and father now have plenty of time to get over the hurt and to proceed with life in what I think of as the normal way.

The emotional and mental side of training in a young athlete's life, especially those like Ron who begin at a terribly early age, can be as destructive as a deterioration of skills. Sports prodigies, like music, art, math, and science prodigies, may lead rewarding lives but those lives are also difficult.

The case of a young ice skater who began serious training at age five is another good example of what can happen to a child and a family.

I didn't meet this skater until she came to me as an adult patient. Her adult problems—insecurity, tentativeness, low self-esteem, introversion—are certainly a result of the traumas of her skating experiences. Like Ron, Betty was considered talented by her parents and was enrolled in private skating lessons at an age when most of her peers were playing with dolls. Betty made solid progress for two years and was thought to be on her way to big things when she began to fail her periodic skating tests. In those days there were eight testing levels recognized by coaches and a youngster who failed more than twice at any of those levels was considered unfit for high-level competition.

Betty made it to level four before she failed and was told obliquely by her coach that she was not likely to do much better in the future. Seeing her chances disappear, she dropped out of the program. Betty told me that later she realized her problem had been more emotional than physical. When she was asked to skate the compulsory figures in her tests she was too nervous to do them properly despite the fact that she had done them perfectly hundreds of times in practice. She told me she still remembers how her legs shook and how she could feel her heart beating hard at those times of stress. She now knows what many top athletes know—that psychological toughness is almost as important as athletic ability when it comes to excellent performance under pressure.

Psychologically speaking, the pressure of competition can motivate or frighten. Some young athletes thrive on it and others can't perform up to their abilities because of it. At least partly, this is because competition requires excellence on command and many youngsters are not capable of combining those two facets of performance. Some athletes simply don't have what society has termed "what it takes" to perform optimally under pressure.

After several months of counseling I determined that most of Betty's adult problems were born on that ice rink more than twenty years earlier. When she recognized this, she was able to put things into perspective and she came to understand that those long-ago failures could be put aside for the business of living as an adult.

I'm not relating these case histories to frighten, only to enlighten. I feel there is something to be learned by all of us from each case.

△ WHAT PARENTS SHOULD DO TO ENCOURAGE SEVEN- TO ELEVEN-YEAR-OLDS △

Let's move on now to what parents can do to sensibly encourage their seven- to eleven-year-old children along the athletic path. Keep in mind that when your child reaches this age he is:

1. Physically capable of throwing, catching, and hitting a ball;

2. Has adequate hand-eye and fine motor coordination;

3. Physically strong enough to participate with most children his age;

4. Mature enough to follow the rules of even the most complicated game.

In short, a seven- to eleven-year-old can play almost any game that an adult can play, especially if modified equipment is available for those children who are small in stature. Also at this age the difference in physical ability between boys and girls is minimal. In fact, the two sexes are more equal during this period

than at any other time, and often a girl will perform at a higher
level than a boy.

But despite this maturing process and the desire you or your
child may have to proceed in a serious and planned way toward
a career in sports, your child:

1. Is not yet emotionally ready to make choices of this nature;

2. Is not intellectually equipped to make these choices;

3. Doesn't know his or her physical capabilities;

4. Will not have reached his or her full potential;

5. Can't be adequately judged by you or by a professional
coach.

It is, therefore, the parents' responsibility to help by making
suggestions and offering options to the child, but not however,
by choosing for the child.

Still, don't be surprised if your child has preferences. You can
convince a six-year-old to go with you to the golf course, but you
may not be able to do the same thing when he reaches seven.
The seven-year-old may also be influenced by his peer group,
which is just fine if his or her friends are engaged in healthy
activities that put the stress on participation rather than
winning.

I've mentioned several times that professional coaching must
be avoided until age twelve or thirteen but that doesn't mean that
the ten-, eleven-, and twelve-year-old can't be introduced to more
organized sports like Little League baseball and Pop Warner football. These leagues are well-established, and though they have
their shortcomings they are generally suitable for most children.
The instruction given in these programs is not regulated, however, so the coach of a given team may be a well-meaning parent
rather than someone knowledgeable in the sport. This isn't necessarily bad, but it does have its drawbacks since a child who
wants informed coaching of some kind may be getting instruction that, if not harmful, may not be helpful either.

For this reason, parents who are more athletically inclined
may want to take on this responsibility themselves by playing
with their child, giving basic instruction, and explaining the
rules of a given sport. Those parents with few athletic skills may
want to arrange for low-pressure lessons for their children with

a coach who is not intent on producing champions. Whenever possible, you should look for lessons that are given in a group format because this too takes the pressure off the individual child. If there are no group lessons available in horse back riding, for example, individual lessons are acceptable if the teacher is carefully chosen and told in advance that you value participation over performance.

Even at this early stage some coaches (even in Little League) will begin to push parents to push their children with such comments as: "Janie rides very well for her age," "I like the way your son throws the ball," and "With a little help, that kid of yours can be a great athlete." This attention may be flattering to your ego, but it shouldn't be taken too seriously. Your child's abilities at this age are subject to fluctuations that no coach can predict. As I have said earlier, growth spurts and hormonal changes affect the athletic ability of a youngster and this in turn affects his or her interests.

The message here is a multifaceted but simple one: Don't put the pressure on to perform, and if you have already done so, take it off. This won't be difficult if you listen to yourself and to your child. The next chapter tells you how to do this.

C H A P T E R

7

△   △

Whose Life Is It, Anyway?

*E*GO IS A powerful drive—so powerful, in fact, that parents often have difficulty distinguishing between the psychological needs of their children and their own personal psychological needs. This is at least partly because human beings have two lives—their real life and their vicarious life. Two case histories will serve to explain this more clearly.

Not long ago I worked with a young girl from Canada whose parents had high hopes for her success as a star in the world of figure skating. At the time, her mother was the stereotypical "back-stage mother," pushy in the extreme. The father was a complacent man who went along with his wife's desires to turn their daughter into an international skating star.

It all started simply enough. In the family's hometown, as in most Canadian towns, ice skating was the sport that everyone took part in. Sarah, like most children in the area, started skating with her parents almost as soon as she was able to walk. It was the natural thing to do and everyone did it.

When she was four, the family skating sessions evolved into Saturday morning classes at the local rink, but for Sarah it was all still recreational and there was no pressure for more instruction from her parents or from Sarah herself. She was small and

△

graceful and she enjoyed the physical activity, the people she skated with, and her parents' attention.

The fact is, Sarah truly liked skating and when she started school she joined an instructional program that met twice a week after school. As she recalls, it was all great fun, she was gaining self-esteem, and the chance to meet other children and to social-ize outside of school was a rewarding experience. And though Sarah didn't show superstar talents, she did seem to have a little more talent than most girls her age.

In Canada, where ice skating is taken seriously, the decision to consider a professional career takes place at an early age. So at age seven, and with a push from her parents, Sarah started competing in formalized Saturday morning figure skating events. She did quite well. At the same time, her parents made the decision to put her on a track that was designed to lead her into a professional skating career. This decision was made after consulting with her instructor but without consulting Sarah.

These critical and far-reaching decisions were made for the child because her parents reasoned:

1. Sarah doesn't know what is best for her.

2. She'll thank us for this later.

3. Sarah, like other children, doesn't have the ability to judge her own talent objectively.

4. This is a great opportunity for all of us.

This line of reasoning leads to the logical conclusion that parents must make this kind of decision for a child.

So at age eight, Sarah's parents enrolled her in a professional training program with a private coach and she began a routine that involved getting up at 5 a.m. each morning in order to get in two hours of skating instruction each day before school. She did not complain and she slowly moved up the ladder in various competitions, though she never did show the kind of exceptional talent necessary to become a professional skater.

Four years later, she reached puberty and went through a number of normal physical changes, but those changes turned the "small and graceful" little girl into a large and ungainly young lady. Her skating progress halted at the same time she was coping with her natural physical changes, and in the eyes of her parents and therefore in her own eyes, her self-esteem dropped rapidly.

Her parents were dismayed at the sudden dip in their daughter's skating fortunes and began to berate her for everything from being lazy to sabotaging all their costly efforts to turn her into a star. She assumed that she was guilty of some gross error and that she had let her parents down. At age thirteen, primarily because of her parents' attitude, Sarah became seriously depressed. She not only dropped out of competitive figure skating but quit skating entirely and had what she described to me as a breakdown. She even had to drop out of school.

When Sarah's parents finally realized the destruction they had caused, they gave up the skating issue and they too became remorseful and felt guilty. The family situation deteriorated so badly that they decided to move from Canada to the United States to avoid the embarrassment the whole incident was causing them in their hometown. That's when they came to see me.

I'm using a sports example here because that is what this book is all about, but exactly the same psychological dynamics are involved when parents make decisions for their children about concentrating their energies in music, art, law, mathematics, medicine, or any other field. Just last year a forty-five-year-old accountant came to me because he was having problems staying on any job for more than eighteen months at a time. This is Jack's story.

As a child, he told me, he was very coordinated and interested in sports, but he was denied the opportunity to participate because his parents wanted him to become a violinist. Both parents were artists: the father a musician and the mother a painter. Both had grown up in a family culture that placed heavy emphasis on academic and artistic achievement. Both parents had struggled in their own professions and had achieved significant successes while still in their early twenties. They met at a concert, courted, and married, and continued their careers for ten more years before deciding to have children.

Their firstborn was a girl who seemed to gravitate naturally to the arts. She was sent to ballet school at age five, the year her brother was born, and she thrived on the discipline demanded by the professional teacher. Of course, she was encouraged at every step by her parents and she made good progress, eventually joining the Royal Ballet of Canada as a student-performer and later as a choreographer.

The parents expected Jack to follow the same predetermined path as the daughter, and as soon as he was old enough to hold a violin they bought him a child-size instrument and sent him off to lessons. The boy had an aptitude for music and he learned quickly. He seemed to enjoy it and often practiced for hours in the privacy of his room. By age eight, Jack had been in several recitals and the parents set their sights on a prestigious competition in Moscow. Their schedule called for him to compete in that contest when he was fifteen, so at age ten they began to enter him in every competition they could find. The boy continued to improve and his teacher told the parents that the boy had the makings of a prodigy. They were thrilled and congratulated themselves on their foresight and good fortune.

Interestingly, Jack had managed to develop athletic skills as well as musical skills and would often sneak off to play basketball or baseball with his friends, either before or after violin lessons. Though he was always fearful of injuring his fingers, he loved sports as much as he loved the violin. It turned out he was quite good in sports as well, but most of all he enjoyed the athletic use of his body and the companionship of peers who were not at all interested in how well he could play the violin.

One afternoon when Jack was fourteen, he told his mother he didn't want to practice the violin any more that day and that he was going out to play ball with his friends. His mother was shocked. She told him in no uncertain terms that he was to practice first and if there was any time left he could play ball. He told her again that he was not going to practice. This defiance so angered the woman that she slapped him with all her strength. He was shocked and frightened and he slapped her back. He then picked up his baseball glove and left the house. That was nearly thirty years ago. Today, though he still likes to listen to music, Jack will not touch an instrument.

When the situation is reversed—that is, when a child is not pressured and chooses to do something on his or her own—it's a different story. Because there is no real problem manifested in such a situation, a psychologist doesn't get cases of this kind, but I will give you an example of that side of the coin from my personal experience.

A few years back, a friend of a friend joined our weekend tennis foursome. Stan's son was fourteen when I met him for the first time. When I got to know him I learned that Stan was a natural athlete, his wife was a former competitive swimmer, and his fourteen-year-old son Joey was a talented tennis player. Stan himself had been a good recreational tennis player as a teenager and was still good though he enjoyed playing just for the fun of it.

As a young boy, Joey had tagged along with his father when he played and the father had always made time to hit the ball with him. Joey was encouraged to play as soon as he showed an interest, but it was not done with a heavy hand. At any rate, Joey got very interested in the game on his own and went through the normal progression of after-school programs, clinics at the park, the two-week tennis camp, and then the six-week tennis camp. It was clear that he liked the sport, but he kept things balanced. He was outgoing, had lots of friends, and liked to play other sports as well as tennis.

When he was fifteen he won the camp tournament in his age group and asked his father if he could go to a professional camp the following summer. Both his parents were encouraging, but they sat him down and asked him the following questions:

1. Are you sure you want to do this?

2. Can you do it without neglecting your other family responsibilities?

3. Can you keep up with your school work?

4. What do you eventually want to do with your tennis?

In other words, they laid out their ground rules as parents and left plenty of room for discussion on Joey's part. He decided he did want to give the camp a try and the next summer he did so.

He finished that summer at the top of his age bracket at the camp, and since his objective was to get a scholarship to one of the good intercollegiate tennis programs, he was well placed to do so. The next year, his last in high school, he was captain of the tennis team and he went on to college as planned.

Joey played tennis well. For him it was good fun and a way to go to college, but it wasn't his whole life and it wasn't the life of his parents either.

△ The Pros and Cons of A Sports Career △

Let's take a closer look at the elements that went into the decisions involving Sarah, Jack, and Joey. First, consider the arguments I hear from parents in favor of a sports career for their children:

1. *Parents know what is best for the child.* I have to agree that parents often do know what's best for their child, especially in the years before the child has developed the ability to make major decisions for himself. Clearly, children need teaching and direction in order to avoid problems parents already understand and know how to solve.

But when it comes to early decisions about careers in sports, music, or whatever, the parent is rarely any better able to make the decision than the child. The facts just aren't there, and when this kind of determination is made it is almost always done to meet the parents' needs and not the needs of the child.

2. *The child will thank his parents later for making this decision.* I've seen far too many cases where the child is more likely to curse his parents than thank them for determining his future before he was old enough to have a say in the decision. In fact, although I've never had such a case, there are many cases cited in the psychological literature that tell of children killing their parents for this very reason. I'm not suggesting that this happens frequently, but it does happen. The point is—don't expect your child to be grateful for fulfilling the dictates of your careful planning, because it is not the norm.

3. *Children don't have the ability to judge their own talent objectively, so parents must do it for them.* It's true that children of ten or eleven aren't good judges of their own talent, but neither are their parents or their coaches. There are just too many factors that enter the picture, not the least of which is the pride parents and coaches take in the performance of their children and their pupils. On the other hand, I've worked with a number of teenagers who were touted as fine athletes but who never fulfilled their potential according to those who made the judgment in the first place. Without exception they've told me they knew at the age of twelve or thirteen that they didn't have it, that they'd seen too many other players who were much better or who had a better temperament for the life of a professional athlete. From my experience I'd have to say that children are perhaps better judges of their abilities than parents and others with an interest strongly invested in their own egos.

4. *A sports career is a great opportunity for us all.* The odds are too great against this argument for a career in sports for it to have any validity. I've cited the statistics elsewhere; they are overwhelming. More likely this great opportunity will turn into a money drain that puts the entire family in a bind and results in recriminations that can affect family relations for years.

Now consider the following questions I know are asked by parents who have doubts about the validity of such a pursuit:

1. *Are you sure you want to do this?* If parents are capable of asking this question, they are parents who have both feet on the ground. When closely questioned, most teenagers will hedge on this point. It makes sense that they aren't sure, not many youngsters are. In fact, an admission of uncertainty is a good indicator that they are candidates for continuing in their training if they desire to do it. People who question their decisions are usually those who have examined them most closely. It's the parents' responsibility to listen to the answer to this question and proceed accordingly.

2. *Can you do it without neglecting your other family responsibilities?* For a teenager, family responsibilities include being a member of the family, not a privileged person who is around from time to time to take meals and receive praise. It means being a part of the regular household routine of chores, family visits, and other social obligations. It means spending time with siblings and acknowledging that the rest of the members of the family are people too.

3. *Can you pay attention to your training and keep up with your school work at the same time?* A surprising number of parents neglect this point. They assume that their athlete in training is not required to spend time on academics and that if he or she needs help the parents or a tutor can take over. But I've interviewed many athletes and most of them have told me something like, "I sure wish I'd paid more attention to my school work." They say this because sports careers are short (they can end at any time—even at age twenty), and because most people athletes meet after their careers are over *aren't* athletes and *are* educated. This is a critical point, and again, it is the responsibility of the parent to see that school is part of the athlete's life.

4. *What do you eventually want to do with your tennis, or golf, or horseback riding, or whatever?* If parents have taken the time to discuss the three previous questions with their youngster, then this question will be easy to answer. In either case, whether to make it a career or a lifetime recreational activity, the answer will be based on reality and a sense that the direction being taken is the right one for the athlete and the family.

What are the overall lessons parents can learn from all of this? The most important is the obvious one: When a child is forced into eight or ten years of what I call "indentured training," there is a high potential for serious problems in the future. This kind of pressure leaves a scar and though a child or a young adult may not murder his parents in their bed because they have forced him to do something he couldn't stand in the end, it is a rare situation in which the child will not eventually impose his own will on his parents and himself. This may take the form of a breakdown as it did with Sarah or open defiance as it did with Jack, but it will eventually surface and may have life-long ramifications.

△ Listen to Your Child △

The other lessons to be learned from the examples of Sarah, Jack, and Joey are not so obvious, or if they seem obvious they are rarely implemented.

1. Parents must be aware that young children do not protest in the same way as adults because they don't have the same verbal weapons as an adult. You can't expect a child with a vocabulary of only a few thousand words to respond to or even understand most of what an adult says. Don't take advantage of your position.

2. A child's mild protests indicate a great deal of dissatisfaction. When a child says, "Let's do it later," or "I don't feel so good," these are really strong protests. The adult equivalents would be "I don't want to do this now or ever," and "The thought of doing this makes me sick to my stomach."

3. Parents must ask the child what he or she wants to do and likes to do. This means not only asking but listening to the

answer. Often when parents ask this kind of question they expect a certain answer and even though that isn't the answer they get, they proceed as if it were. So, for example, you may find yourself asking your youngster: "Do you want to play catch?" and getting a firm "no" for an answer. If you've been listening you might say, "Why not?" or "Okay," but since it's your idea you may answer, "Great, let's go." Ask, and then listen.

4. The child's reasons for wanting or refusing to do something must be explored. As adults, we shouldn't be turned away by a negative answer. If a child doesn't want to do something, there is probably more than one reason including another idea, tiredness, boredom, sickness, hunger, or fear. Consider these possible reasons and try to figure out which ones are valid at the time. It can help you in making future approaches.

△ Examine Your Own Motives △

What it boils down to is this: It is the child's needs that count, not those of the parent or parents. Thus, as it should be, *the onus is on the parent to determine his or her own needs and motivations for putting a child into any form of professional training.* The parent must be able to judge if he or she is living vicariously through the child and be prepared to face the reality that just such a thing is possible. It isn't an easy thing to do because it requires a close and potentially hurtful self-examination.

Don't get me wrong. There is nothing intrinsically wrong with vicarious experiences. But when that experience comes at the expense of the child (and usually other members of the family as well), the price is too high. One of the reasons we have children to begin with is to have the satisfaction of living vicariously through the child, and parents can still have that gratification without forcing the child to be a better version of themselves.

The first question a parent should ask himself or herself is, "What are my own needs and why do I want my child to be involved in sports (or music or dance, etc.)?" Here are some other questions to ask yourself:

1. Do I want this because it's good for my child's physical and emotional development?

2. Do I want it because then my child will be able to share something with me?

3. Do I want it because my child is expressing a need to participate?

4. Do I want it because it will make me proud of him or her if he or she does well?

5. Do I want it because I did it and that will make my child more like me?

6. Do I want it because my child is an extension of me and I can increase my own value and self-worth through his or her performance?

7. Do I want it because if my child is successful, he or she will make a lot of money and take care of me in my retirement?

Let's look at the possible answers to these questions and their importance:

1. If the answer is yes, then you're on the right track. If the answer is no, then you must figure out why you do want it. The answer to some of the following questions will give you an idea of what your reasons really are.

2. There is nothing wrong with a yes answer here. Sharing with your child is an admirable idea. If the answer is no, then there are some other reasons that need to be uncovered.

3. If your child is expressing a need to participate in sports or a particular sport, that's fine. If it seems that it is your needs that are being expressed, you must look closely at the reasons why.

4. Parental pride is a marvelous thing, but it shouldn't be based on the quality of your child's performance. Just being on a team or playing in a tournament takes guts and some talent. Recognize this and try and separate it from the fact that you would be pleased if that performance was also of star quality.

5. If you played baseball and you want your child to play baseball, that's fine. Be careful, however, that the decision to play

baseball is made by the child and not by you for your own reasons.

6. This is very likely a reason for wanting your child to have a career in sports. Your child is an extension of you and you *can* increase your own self-worth through the child's performance, but again, the pressure is being put on the child to perform in order to enhance your self-worth. This isn't a fair exchange.

7. Believe it or not, this is a reason that many people give for wanting a sports career for their child. It has no psychological validity and very little social validity, but it is a consideration. Parents often make the personal sacrifices and the investment in training not so much for their child's future but for their own.

As a child gets older, the potential for parents to apply pressure is greater, especially if the youngster shows some talent. The key element for parents to recognize is that a parents' desires can be, and often are, a function of his or her own lack of self-esteem and need to live vicariously and experience excellence through the performance of the child.

The parent who feels secure, competent, and adequate in the world isn't going to do that to a child. If it's a sports career the parents want, the opportunity is there to begin applying the pressure as soon as a child starts to crawl. You can experience vicarious pleasure very quickly because you can watch the child perform the tasks in miniature that you envision for him later.

Here's one final case history that once again illustrates the impact of parental pressure.

Two athletic parents, the father a fine amateur tennis player and the mother a professional golfer, decided that their daughter, an only child, should become a professional golfer. At age nine, they sent the girl to a professional golf camp where she played golf all day and studied with private tutors during the evening. She was a good player for her age but had little competitive fire. Besides, she was more interested in her school work, especially literature, than in playing golf.

At one point the coach met with the parents to tell them that the daughter was a more than adequate player and showed the talent to be an exceptional player but that unless she committed herself more completely to her game she was just going to be a good player who'd win age-group tournaments until she was twelve or thirteen and after that the really good players would start to beat her rather easily.

The parents had a long talk with the girl as they walked around the golf course, and she told them very clearly that she enjoyed the game and some of the people but that she was more interested in going to a regular school with regular children than she was in golf. The parents insisted that this was nonsense and that she would continue whether she wanted to or not. Though this conversation left the girl in tears the parents were satisfied that they had done the right thing and that the daughter had gotten the message.

Almost immediately after that the girl developed an eating disorder and began to lose weight. As she lost strength and stamina, her golf game deteriorated and as she realized that she was not pleasing her parents she became gradually more depressed. The coach called the parents and told them of the situation, but they assured him that she would come out of it. Four days later the girl swam out to the middle of the lake at the golf camp and let herself sink to the bottom.

Again, I'm not telling this story to frighten parents. But it would be silly to write a book on this subject without presenting all the potential ramifications of parents trying to live vicariously through the sports exploits of their children.

CHAPTER

8

△ △

Making the Big Decision

*T*HE RULES OF the game start to change when a young person reaches the age of twelve. It is at this age, give or take a year, that a talented youngster and his or her family come to a place where the athletic road divides into two forks.

One of these forks leads toward what I would call a "normal" relationship with sports—that is, a desire to play a game or several games well, to have fun, and to make sports an integral, but not a central, part of life.

The other fork leads toward a "serious" commitment to sports in which the ultimate goal may be playing a given sport for international recognition in such events as the Olympics or for financial gain in the world of professional sports. In short, this fork means making a career in sports.

The fork that leads to sports for fun and fitness is obviously the most common one. But for youngsters with a degree of talent it is no less difficult to decide that sports will not be a professional career choice than it is for a youngster with talent who decides to follow the fork that leads to a serious commitment to a career in sports. The fact is, in many instances it is a good deal harder for a talented youngster to step back from his or her involvement far enough to look at all the effort that has been

△

expended and accept the fact that all it adds up to is the compilation of skills that may lead to some future time spent in an enjoyable pastime.

For example, a young gymnast with better than average ability, a youngster who enjoys the excitement, the competition, the camaraderie, the attention, and the exercise provided by the sport has already made a tremendous investment in time and energy (and probably money as well) by age twelve. There is bound to be an ambivalence about a decision not to continue, not only because of this considerable investment but also because it means "never giving it a shot"—that is, never testing the full measure of his or her ability. In many cases, this is often the point in life where a youngster sets the stage for his or her first serious regrets; the spot that he or she may look back on years later and say, "I should at least have tried."

Be that as it may, the factors used to make the decision to pursue sports toward a career goal or to stop in that pursuit are essentially the same for the athlete and his or her family. And the critical family decision that must be made at this time cannot be made in a vacuum or in haste. Here are the issues that are involved in making that decision:

▷ An assessment of the odds

▷ The actual talents of the child

▷ The desire of the child

▷ The desire of the parents

▷ The commitment of the parents

▷ The place of siblings in the picture

▷ The financial costs

▷ The time involved

▷ The emotional consequences

▷ The potential for success

▷ The possibility of failure

▷ The real rewards

▷ The imagined rewards

▷ The unforeseen

▷ The life after sports

The problem, of course, is how to weigh and assess all of these issues as objectively as possible when objectivity is in short supply. How does a parent objectively judge if his youngster has the ability to pursue a sports career that could lead to the Olympics, or to a college scholarship, and eventually to a contract with a professional team? This evaluation is extremely difficult for an outsider like a coach, let alone for a parent. How does a parent objectively judge whether the family can and should support this effort? How does a family estimate the costs of such a commitment?

Families who have reached this fork in the road have surely talked in general about these questions, but in my experience, it is the rare family that has taken the time to explore them in any depth. Let's consider the principal issues here.

△ Judging the Odds △

First let's look at a hard reality that affects even the most talented athlete—the extremely heavy odds against success as a college athlete, an Olympian, and a professional.

Though all of the points listed above are critical, perhaps the most important, and the most neglected, is making an honest assessment of the odds against any youngster attaining world-class status in any sport—amateur or professional. This is an assessment that should be based on hard numbers as well as psychological considerations, and it should be made before the fact, not after serious training has begun.

The professional athlete, with a few exceptions, must endure years of training, pass through an extended period of what might be called apprenticeship—either in college, in sponsored competitions at various levels, or in the minor leagues as is the practice in baseball. This is an absolute prerequisite before there is any opportunity at all in the professional ranks. Today's competition is fierce and the days are gone when a youngster can walk onto the field cold and have a chance to make the team regardless of his or her raw talent.

There are more than two million high school athletes, and if you recall the number of good athletes on your various high school teams you can see that the competition for places on college athletic squads, and for scholarships, is intense.

Out of that pool of two million athletes, the country's colleges give athletic scholarships to an estimated 20,000 young men and women. Many of these superb athletes play good—even great—football, basketball, baseball, or whatever. After three or four years of competition, several thousand of these athletes, both the good and the very good, have dropped out of contention for the pros or the Olympics because of injury, a decision to play out the college string and not go on, plans for further schooling, a loss of interest during their college years, or a realization that, compared to their peers, they really don't have the talent to go any further. Nevertheless, a good number of college athletes (as many as 10,000 each year) continue to harbor the dream of a professional career and pursue that dream with vigor. Upon graduation, they have high hopes that a sports career lies ahead of them.

Most of those dreams are quickly shattered, simply because there are not enough places to work. In this country, there are roughly 2,000 jobs available in the four major spectator sports of baseball, football, basketball, and hockey. There are approximately 500 more spots in tournament time golf and tennis, and a few more in soccer, ice skating, and running. So if we're generous we can say there are 3,000 people who are bona fide professional athletes, that is, people whose primary job is performing in front of public. Of these, 1,500 or so earn a lot of money, another 500 earn substantial money, and the rest earn a living. But that's not the whole story.

There may be 3,000 potential jobs overall, but each year there are only a few positions available on any given team and fewer jobs still on the tennis and golf circuit. The worlds of international gymnastics, track and field, ice skating, and soccer add only a handful more jobs to the pool.

Breaking it down even further, the average number of rookie players who make one of the 26 professional football squads each year is less than four, and only one of those will go on to become a star player making big money. The story is just about the same in baseball and hockey, and it is much lower in basketball, where teams have only ten players each. Sure, there is the occasional rookie player who signs a contract for $1 million, but they are rare birds. Most rookies get a small signing bonus and the mini-mum salary and then labor in the vineyards until they become established players or decide to find other work. As you can read-ily see, the odds are not good.

There is one other point that must be made here. Sports careers are short. The professional life expectancy of the average professional football player is three years; in basketball it is four, in baseball, five. And consider the fact that since the big names in all sports play for ten or twelve years, the terms of their careers tend to increase the average for all the other players. The longev-ity of Pete Rose, Joe Montana, Jimmy Conners, and Jack Nicklaus is far from the norm.

The message here is clear: Dont' delude yourself as a parent and even more important, don't delude your youngster about the prospects of a life in professional sports. The odds are not the kind you would want to bet on.

I know this recital of facts about the reality of a career in sports isn't likely to change anyone's mind, but I would be remiss if I didn't point out the dangers of overconfidence, because such delusions of grandeur can create serious, long-range repercus-sions for an athlete and his family.

I currently have a patient who at age fifty-one is still suffering because his plans for a career in professional baseball never materialized. Stan grew up in the Midwest and though he was not a big person he was extremely well coordinated. He played all sports well, and was the kind of youngster who could pick up a golf club or a tennis racket for the first time and play quite an acceptable game. When he was twelve years old he was only 5' 3" and wore thick glasses, but it was that year that he decided he was going to be a professional baseball player.

Stan's parents encouraged him to play, but his father was quick to tell the boy that he thought there were other things he might want to consider doing in life. In retrospect, Stan now knows that his father was telling him in a nice way that even though he was a good ballplayer, in the long run he wasn't really going to be able to compete against bigger and stronger players.

Still Stan persevered. He was bright and understood that because of his weak eyesight he was not going to be a great hit-ter, so he concentrated on pitching and catching and was good at both. He spent every waking hour playing in the various leagues in his town, sometimes playing three games in one day by pitching in one and catching in the other two.

All through high school he prepared himself for a baseball career, and when all of his friends started making plans for college, he made plans to sign a baseball contract and leave college for another time. Stan's father wasn't particularly happy about this decision but went along with it thinking the boy would soon come face to face with reality. At seventeen, the boy signed a minor league contract with a New York Yankee farm team and as his friends finished their last year of high school and prepared for college he went off to spring training in Florida. The experience turned out to be the happiest and saddest time of Stan's life because after three weeks he was cut from the team.

He now remembers that he saw it coming. As he watched his competition he knew that though he was good, he wasn't in the same class as most of the rookies in camp. When the cut came he was not surprised, but he was depressed, and he packed his bags and went back to his home. Stan's parents were exceptionally understanding and sensitive to his situation and urged him to go to summer school to finish up his last year of high school and to go on to college like his friends.

But the young man was too depressed to follow their sensible suggestion. Rather than see his old friends and face up to the razzing he thought he'd receive, he withdrew. He spent long hours in that hot summer in his room doing little more than listening to the radio. His friends would call but he didn't want to talk with them so they soon stopped bothering to get in touch. His depression got so deep that he stopped eating and almost never left his room. His parents, deeply concerned since his return, became desperate. They were finally able to get him to see a psychologist but that had little effect.

Finally, at age twenty-three Stan went into the army and though he wasn't particularly happy there, he was able to play on the post baseball team and he made quite a name for himself as an army all-star. He stayed in the army and later became the manager of a team that won the armed services baseball championship. After twenty-five years he left the service and that's when he came to me.

He is searching for something to do with the rest of his life and we are hard at work on that problem. Two years ago he enrolled in a local college and is working toward a degree in law, which is a positive step. But he still has severe bouts of depression and those must be overcome if he is to lead a normal and productive life from this point on. I have high hopes for this man, but his future is uncertain.

The possibility of failure and the need for alternative plans.
Stan's case highlights some of the psychological considerations
that are involved on both sides of the decision to follow a career
in sports. Not only does the youngster have to be aware of the
very real possibility of failure and, further, understand that it is
the norm rather than the exception, but he or she should be
strongly advised to make alternate plans should their choice of a
sports career not work out or should injury curtail further
competition.

As I've said throughout this book, this is the parent's responsibility. Young people do not have the life experience or the judgment to foresee the potential for failure and to act to mitigate its
potentially disastrous results.

Stan's case also points out the fact that even the most concerned parent can't control a young adult's life if the youngster
is firmly commited to a given course. But the effort must be
made in order to fulfill your obligations as a parent.

△ Judging Your Child's Talent △

With rare exceptions, parents are not able to accurately discriminate when it comes to their own child's talent. (In fact, in my
experience it is more often the youngster who is the best judge
of his or her own talent and not parents, coaches, or other outsid-
ers.) The parents' clear vision is often obscured because they
have so much invested in the entire parenting process they can't
separate wishes—their own or their child's—from reality.

In fact, the decision about the extent of a youngster's talent—
whether it's the ability to hit a baseball, throw a football, ride a
horse, paint a picture, write a story, or play an instrument—is
often made by the parents long before the child displays much
in the way of real talent in any particular area. Sometimes, and
I have worked with such cases, the decision is made before the
child is born. Everything that occurs after that becomes a self-
fulfilling prophecy.

Parents certainly have the greatest vested interest in their
child-athlete, but coaches—from Little League through high
school and college—develop a vested interest as well. A good athlete gives a coach a special aura, and nurturing that athlete's

particular talent can become an obsession because of the obvious psychic rewards the coach receives. The coach may also receive monetary rewards as well because a very gifted athlete reflects favorably on the coach who, as a result of his real or perceived effect on the athlete, may get a job at a bigger school or become the athlete's mentor or even his agent.

Let's take a closer look at the questions, problems, and pitfalls involved in the evaluation of talent by reviewing some case histories.

The following story was revealed to me by a recent patient, Pat, a boy of twelve from an upper middle class family. The father in this case was a thirty-six-year-old man who had played tennis since he was a child and though he played well enough to compete with his friends, he was never a top-flight player. As soon as his son Pat was old enough, the father started playing tennis with him and found the boy to be well-coordinated and athletic. To the father, the boy had seemed genuinely interested in tennis, but as soon as I talked with him it was clear that a good part of the emotional reward Pat was getting from playing was the loving approval of his parents, especially his father. It was also clear that Pat was worried that he would lose his father's love if he stopped playing or didn't play well enough.

By the time Pat was seven the father's objectivity had disappeared and his wishful thinking had taken over. It was at that time that Pat's father started entering his son in local and area tournaments. He was good enough to win many of them and when he didn't win he usually finished among the top four. Because both father and son were interested in tennis, the father took Pat to many tennis events that were held relatively nearby, and to major professional tournaments in other cities. For Pat, this not only offered a chance to watch tennis stars in action, but more importantly, a chance to spend time with his father and to share a special experience with his dad.

The fact is, the boy did enjoy playing and watching tennis to a certain extent, but mostly he liked the idea and the feeling of sharing things with his father and receiving his father's attention and approval. Though his mother encouraged his interest in tennis, she was less enthusiastic than her husband. But to a large extent Pat tried to excel in order to please both his parents and make them proud of him. (By the way, this is typical. It is usually one parent, either mother or father, who is involved in actively encouraging a child when it comes to an interest in sports.)

When Pat was age ten, the father, with his son's acquiescence (he could hardly say no), decided it was time for the boy to go to a professional tennis camp for the summer. The one chosen by the father was a prestigious camp about four hours from the family home. Pat had received a recommendation from his coach at home and the camp director, a former professional, was glad to accept Pat in the program based on that recommendation.

Halfway through that summer, Pat's parents came up to visit him and the discovery made by the father on that visit was the basis for a serious family crisis. The cause of the problem was the news Pat's parents received from the camp director just after their arrival. The director told them that through his own observations and those of the teaching staff, it had been determined that Pat was a good tennis player for his age, but that he was not an exceptional player and certainly didn't have the talent to compete with other good players his age. He went on to say that it was possible that Pat was a little above average for ten-year-olds in his area, but when thrown in with his counterparts from around the country, he was very much in the middle—in short, a slightly above average player. He went on to tell the parents that Pat might be good enough to make his high school team and that he would always be a good recreational player if he so chose, but that it would not be a good idea to send him to a specialty camp again. The director was candid in saying that "it was a waste of money" for Pat to spend any more time in professional training.

The head of the program—a sophisticated and sensitive man—expressed his concern to Pat's parents before they saw the boy because he had seen how important the camp was to Pat and, through Pat's comments, how much he was worried about his parents' reaction to his progress or lack of it. Pat had showed signs of anxiety about his level of performance and his own recognition that he wasn't as good as his dad thought he was. The director told the parents about Pat's reactions and cautioned the father not to come down on the boy, because it certainly wasn't his fault that he wasn't a great player. He might have added, but didn't, that it wasn't the boy's fault that his father wanted him to be a tennis star either.

Though the father may have privately suspected that his son was not a great player, getting the facts about his son's talents from a trained professional was something the father wasn't prepared for. He immediately began to deny the facts with remarks to the coach like, "Pat needs more time to show his best stuff," "I've seen what he can do," and "He may need more private lessons, but he has the potential." He went on to tell the program director that he was probably wrong in his assessment of Pat and that he had felt "there was a certain animosity toward my son when we arrived."

To his son, the father was neither supportive nor encouraging, and he offered none of the parental warmth that the child desperately needed at that time. He volunteered nothing in the way of loving words or gestures and this added to the boy's profound feeling of inadequacy and guilt at having let his father down.

The parents left the camp early, not even bothering to stay for the entire weekend, and Pat finished out the summer in something of a daze. Quite understandably, his tennis got worse instead of better.

When he returned home at the end of the summer the situation had hardened with the father, and the mother was no help at all because she was having difficulty justifying her behavior throughout the entire episode. Pat was already distraught when he got home, but the situation quickly became worse when he found his father was so unforgiving. He could draw no other conclusion except that he let his dad down and that he had somehow failed personally. And he had no one to talk to about his concerns because neither of his parents were able to approach the subject without recriminations.

When they were referred to me by a mutual friend, I found the whole family in shambles. The boy was depressed, he had lost weight, and he was doing poorly in school. The parents were fighting with each other, the wife was having an affair, and the couple was about to separate.

The boy's father had been shattered by the boy's failure, which he internalized to mean his own failure. What he had expected was his son's triumph, which would have taken care of his vicarious need for fulfillment in sports. The boy was destroyed because he had failed, and the mother was angry with the father because of his attitude and her inability to intercede effectively between father and son.

As bad as the situation was, the father could have done worse. For example, he could have continued to berate his son or he could have insisted that he go to another camp where people wouldn't "have it in for him," or he could have ignored the situation entirely and dismissed the boy as hopeless. Fortunately, however, he didn't compound the problem with any of these reactions, and he did respond when our mutual friend suggested therapy.

It was a painful and chaotic time for the entire family and it took a year of family therapy to mend the worst of the wounds, establish a dialogue between father and son, bring the mother back into the picture, and put things in general into perspective.

Pat finally understood and accepted the fact that his father was disappointed and the father was again able to express his love for the boy without reservations. The father was also able to recognize that it had been his own desire—part of his unfulfilled and previously unexpressed dreams of playing professional tennis—and not that of his son, to have the boy invest his time and energy in playing tennis seriously. In essence, the father took the pressure off. And the mother, who had opted out of the situation and was angered by her inability to participate, was finally able to express her feelings to her husband about his attitude and approach to their son and to her.

Father and son even started to play tennis again, but the boy soon drifted off to play with his friends and gave up competing entirely because he had found that it was fun to play for the pleasure of playing and difficult to play under pressure.

You can see from this example that it isn't only numerical odds that stack up against a youngster who wants to (or is convinced to) follow a career path in sports. Early evaluations are tough judgment calls and, as a parent, you have to be fully prepared for those judgments to be wrong. A teenager can be carefully groomed for a career in sports and still not make it for any number of reasons, but lack of sufficient talent is the single most important factor in the final analysis.

Clearly, failure must be considered, even expected, and this too must be acknowledged in the beginning by both the parents and their child. Life plans should not be based on being on the tennis circuit or playing pro baseball or winning the Olympic pole vault. If that's how it turns out, the necessary adjustments can be made. Parents, beware of maintaining that your child "has the right stuff" or "we're going to do it or die trying." This kind of approach is something like going to a horse race and betting on the long shot. I'm not saying you shouldn't bet on that horse, but when you do, don't kid yourself about your chances and don't bet more than you can afford to lose. In short, don't put more into the effort of making your child a success in sports than you're prepared to lose.

The following case illustrates the consequences of betting more financially and emotionally than one family was prepared to lose.

I have been interested in horses all my life, but I didn't take up riding seriously until I was an adult. Then I threw myself into it wholeheartedly and eventually reached a skill level where I could compete in horse shows and even win ribbons.

Five years ago I met a well-to-do New York family at one of the area's shows. In the course of the conversation they mentioned that their daughter was also competing and that they would like me to meet her. I did meet her and six months later she and the family became patients of mine.

Here is the story. The girl, whose name is Karen, had started riding when she was eight, not because her parents were avid horsemen but because one of her friends was taking lessons and it all sounded like great fun. Karen started as most children start, by taking lessons once a week at a stable that offered instruction and small horses. She showed some ability, which thrilled her parents, and within six months they made a commitment to her progress by buying her a pony of her own.

The following year Karen started competing in sanctioned horse shows and by the time she was twelve she had moved up in class from ponies to full-size horses. She won a few ribbons in the local shows and her parents made the next move: they bought her an expensive horse; in this case, a horse with a price tag of $40,000. Now she was taking lessons every day after school at the stables and going to out-of-town shows and competing on the weekends. This represented a considerable investment for her parents—paying board for the horse at $1,000 a month, paying the coach $150 a week, fees for entering the shows, trucking fees for the horse, and their own expenses as they traveled from show to show. The total cost of Karen's involvement had risen to nearly $25,000 a year, not counting the cost of the horse.

This had turned into the parents' pursuit of an athletic career for Karen, not because they found her progress so exciting but because they enjoyed all of the social ramifications that are part of the world of horse shows. For the parents the main attraction of all of this was the entrée it gave them into the horsey set and a social circle that they wanted to be part of. For them it meant rubbing elbows with the rich, it meant horse shows and fashion shows, cocktail parties, formal dinners, and charity balls. The parents were getting a lot of mileage out of it all.

Then things started to go downhill. It wasn't that the family couldn't afford it, that was the easy part, but Karen was now struggling with school because she was at the stable every afternoon. All her friends were girls who rode with her and she was included in all the social events her parents attended, even though she would rather have been elsewhere. Things began to come unraveled when she was fifteen and discovered boys. Immediately, she became less interested in riding and more interested in hanging out at the local pizza parlor with her new-found boy friends.

Her parents got very upset with the turn of events and she was severely chastised by her father, who said in essence: "You've got seven years of time invested in riding, we've invested tens of thousands of dollars in lessons, camps, horses, etc., and now you want to hang out, eat pizza, and go to rock concerts because Johnny Jones is a cute kid. You're letting us down."

That's when they came to me. After several sessions it became clear that Karen's mother was much more involved in the social aspects of Karen's riding career than in the riding itself—much more than even she realized. She had also been more intimately involved with the mechanics of Karen's life, as mothers usually are. She had been responsible for driving Karen to and from the stable, had comforted her daughter when she was not riding well and when she lost in the shows, and she was the one who sympathized when she fell and when her horse was injured. The father was more the proud observer of his daughter's accomplishments. He enjoyed the shows and the company of other successful men and women, and he liked sipping champagne with the uppercrust. But it was the mother who was really invested: Her whole social circle was built around the trips to horse shows, horse auctions, and charity events.

Karen's decision to eat pizza instead of sip champagne precipitated the final stage of the family crisis. The mother tried bribing Karen to continue, she threatened, she cajoled. Nothing worked, and as a result of all the pressure, Karen went on a spree of drinking, eating, and keeping late hours. Her mother went into a state of depression.

Fortunately, Karen was strong-willed and she quickly pulled herself out of her funk. After only a few weeks she was back on her feet. Not so with her mother. The woman continued in a depressed state for two years. During this period the husband met and had an affair with another woman and the couple is now divorced.

Karen, however, is living with her father, has given up riding, improved her school performance, and is planning on entering college next year.

There are four valuable lessons to be learned from the examples of Pat and Karen:

1. The sooner a young person's talent is evaluated the better.

2. Regardless of whether the evaluation is negative or positive, it must be listened to and adhered to.

3. A parent's desires must not be imposed upon the child.

4. The parent is ultimately responsible for the child's well-being.

Of course, there were positive aspects in these experiences for the families involved. First, they found out early enough that their children didn't have the exceptional ability necessary to pursue a sports career or that the inclination was lacking, or both. This saved them from having to face the same problem, only magnified by the adolescent years, when Pat and Karen reached their late teens. They also had the sense to recognize that sports had caused a major problem within the family and to see that they needed outside help to solve that problem.

In Pat's case, the father was eventually able to accept and follow the recommendation of the tennis camp director that he not continue to push his son to excel when the boy's skills were only average.

And here credit must go to the camp director, because he had the ethics and the courage to be straightforward with Pat's parents. This is not always the case. I have met many parents who have been led by professional camp directors to belive that their children had exceptional talent when they did not. Unfortunately, this is done primarily because a camp is a business and a business needs customers.

As we have seen, it's quite common for parents to use their children as surrogates to achieve some life goal that has long since been out of reach. Essentially, the parent is living through the child's performance, finally filling that void left by some unachieved goal in their own lives. There is a direct correlation between the parent's own self-esteem, or lack of it, and the need to impose their own desires on their child. The parent who feels secure and competent isn't going to do what Pat's father did.

Parents' obsessive need for the child to excel affect other areas of a child's life as well. I have young people in my practice who are experiencing exactly the same kind of parental pressure only it is pressure to perform in school. Their parents are driving them to be excellent even though there is no particular educational goal in mind except that ephemeral long-term goal of getting into a good university. Of course, to do that there are interim goals that parents perceive and set, and the first one is often to get their child into the "right" nursery school. This is supposed to lead to the "right" elementary or private school, then the "right" high school or prep school, and ultimately to the "right" university.

These interim goals are also imposed when it comes to sports, so that it becomes important that a child progress from a good peewee baseball team to a good Little League team, that they qualify to make the annual trip to play in another town, and so on. If you see yourself entangled in this upward spiral, you are not alone.

But look at the other side of the coin for just a moment. More successful youngsters come from families where the parents don't continually drive their children and where the parental goal is to produce normal, healthy human beings. Sure, children in these families are encouraged to do well and to test themselves, but at the same time they are helped to work within their own abilities.

Finally, parents must recognize with complete clarity that they are ultimately responsible for their child's well-being. That means, as in the case of Pat, accepting the professional opinion of the tennis coach, but more than that, it means accepting the fact that your own desires are secondary to those of the child and that the imposition of pressure can more often be destructive than helpful.

Second opinions. The case of Pat and the tennis camp also raises another question. Should parents, faced with a negative evaluation of the skills of their child seek a "second opinion," as they might do in a medical situation? Many parents are surprisingly willing to go from coach to coach, camp to camp, and to fly all over the country to seek out the opinion they want. It is not only expensive to pursue this course, but it can be a never-ending quest for the Holy Grail. After one negative and one positive evaluation, for example, it's almost imperative that you get a third appraisal. If the third is negative, then a fourth is in order and so on. So I say no to a second opinion if the first one is strongly negative or overwhelmingly positive. But when the first opinion is moderately positive or praiseworthy, I think it's a good idea to get more advice.

As I said, professional camps, especially specialty camps, are in business to make money, and it's an unfortunate fact that some of them are not above giving false hope to parents intent on the success of their child. Parents with that intent are easily deluded into believing that their child has exceptional ability. Camp directors will use phrases like, "He made a lot of progress this summer" and "She has tremendous potential." These expressions of modest praise are causes for concern rather than celebration. Neither of these mildly encouraging comments or others like them, pin the issue down. And the reality, that of the youngster's true level of talent, can be obscured. Of course, the parent cannot make these distinctions if he has lost track of the boundaries between his own needs and those of the child. There is no way to objectively guide, monitor, or counsel if you're totally involved.

△ Judging Your Child's (and Your Own) Desire △

The critical element of the story about Pat and his family is the one that never happened. The parents, especially the father, should have had a serious talk with Pat to determine what Pat himself wanted to do long before he was sent to camp. In this case, it is likely that Pat would have gone along with his father's plan because he was so intent on pleasing him, but just possibly Pat might have said something to indicate his true feelings. This goes back to the point that the child's desires are the critical factor, and his or her opinions must be solicited and listened to as well. In this case, Pat's desire to play tennis was not organic— that is, it didn't grow out of his own interests and ability but out of his father's needs and his desire to please his father.

To determine your child's desire, you must establish a dialogue with him. I know that establishing a dialogue with anyone is often something that is easier said than done. Neither individuals, nor spouses, nor children seem well disposed to the concept of open discussion. Moreover, there are no established rules for going about this sensitive task in our society; certainly no single way of doing it. Still, it is a crucial practice. Perhaps the most critical element of such a dialogue is that the parent first take a hard look at himself to determine his own motivations. This takes some honest exploration. I have listed some important questions for parents to ask themselves about why they want their child to be involved in sports.

1. Is it because it will be good for my child's physical development?

2. Is it because it will be good for my child's emotional development?

3. Is it so my child will be able to share something with me or vice versa?

4. Is it because my child is expressing a need to participate?

5. Is it because it will make me proud of my child if he or she does well?

6. Is it because I did it and it will make my child more like me?

7. Is it because I can increase my own self-esteem by my child's participation?

8. Is it because my child's success can mean money and security for the family?

Talking with your child won't be easy, but it may be somewhat easier than questioning yourself. Begin by making a list of some of the things you know about your child. Here are some factors to consider:

▷ Is he verbal and outgoing or non-verbal and private?

▷ Is he generally assertive or apprehensive and fearful?

▷ Does he have a sense of humor or is it hard to joke with him?

▷ Is he sensitive or insensitive?

▷ Is he motivated or unmotivated?

▷ Does he seek approval or not care about approval?

▷ Is he competitive or noncompetitive?

▷ Is he physically active or sedentary?

Next, decide which spouse is the primary communicator in the family. If one or the other has a better rapport with the child, then that spouse should be the one to do most of the talking. If both spouses have equal levels of communication with the child, then both should be involved. And even if one spouse acts as the primary spokesman, the other should be present and included in the conversation even if it's only as an observer.

When should this discussion take place? This depends on previously established family patterns. Ask yourself these questions:

1. Where does most of the family's conversation take place? Is it around the dinner table or is it after dinner or some other time when the family is together?

2. Are issues of parenting discussed as an on-going part of family life, or do such discussions take place around specific issues such as a bad report card or a fight with a neighbor or sibling?

3. Are feelings easily expressed in your family, or do family members generally suppress their feelings?

4. Does family interaction take place naturally and easily, or does it have to be forced?

The answers to these questions will give you an idea of what is called the "family dynamic," but more importantly it will tell you when and how to hold a dialogue around the issue of sports participation—or around any other issue of importance to the entire family.

Of course, you don't need to immobilize yourself while you wait for all the planets to become properly aligned. As a general rule, all matters of parental and family concern are better addressed in the course of the normal family routine than set aside as a special conference, because this automatically makes them a larger issue. There has been a lot written and said about the value of a regular, or even an irregular, "family meeting" to discuss important issues. This sounds good, but in my experience it rarely works well. So try to avoid saying something like, "Saturday at two o'clock we're all going to sit down and talk about this matter of Jenny's participation in sports." Let it happen naturally, or at least plan it so that it seems to occur spontaneously.

A particular crisis situation, however, needs to be addressed directly and immediately. For example, if you're playing catch with your son and he has a temper tantrum, starts throwing his glove, and yelling obscenities, immediate action is necessary. The impact of your feelings and opinions will be lost if you say, "Johnny, we're going to have a serious talk about this later." Some things can't be set aside for later.

This doesn't mean you have to hold a tight reign on your child. Emotion is fine. Venting frustration is normal. But children need a structure that sets out acceptable limits and when those limits are exceeded, parental action is demanded. If behavior is radically outside the norm, it has to be dealt with on the spot. The alternative can result in the creation of a temperamental monster who is outside everyone's control.

So if you get a call from the Little League coach (or the math teacher or the music instructor) saying that your son threw his helmet three times at the last practice and in general was acting like a little jerk, act on this information. Depending on your child, this confrontation may be easy or difficult, but it can't be allowed to go unnoticed.

It's interesting that sometimes these types of problems seem special because they are sports-connected. They really aren't out of the ordinary, only a part of the whole parenting process.

Talking About Feelings

Our American society does not put a high premium on openly expressing personal feelings. In fact, it's just the opposite, especially for young boys and men. The message American society gives in general is, "Shut up and get on with it." Negative feelings such as anger, pain, and sadness are considered especially inappropriate.

What this means is that a youngster can come home and proudly announce that he hit a home run but fail to mention that he also made four errors and could use a hug. Since our youngsters are not apt to tell us these things, we must know them well enough to see or suspect that things aren't exactly right.

Here are some techniques to use with youngsters who have trouble making their feelings known:

1. Get into the habit of talking to your child about things in general.

2. Establish the practice of talking about feelings and experiences whenever it's natural so that on the occasions when it's necessary it won't seem like something out of the ordinary.

3. Talk about your own difficult experiences and disappointments when appropriate.

The talking habit is contagious. It isn't at all necessary that every conversation have a specific topic, such as homework or household chores. Conversations with children should be very much like conversations with adults—open-ended and free-flowing with interjections and interruptions, opinions, agreements and disagreements, give and take.

Talking about feelings is a different story. In many families, feelings are suppressed and kept private and any interaction on the subject is forced rather than natural. In that kind of family, it is important for the parents to recognize that there is difficulty in this area and take advantage of the help that is available in facilitating this kind of family communication.

Again, you have to do some honest evaluation. If communication about feelings in your family is not open and you kid yourself into thinking it is, you're only cheating yourself and your family.

I could give some stock advice here on how to open these intra-family communications, but the reality is that the absence of this kind of family dynamic is a complex matter and doesn't give in easily to a stock approach. The problem is generally that the personalities in a particular family don't interact well. In this case, the problem for these people is not limited to family situations alone. They don't communicate well in social contexts outside of the family either. This doesn't mean these noncommunicative people are "sick." They may simply be reserved or not have developed good communications skills because their parents didn't have them and they weren't exposed to them. However, with the help of a facilitator—a psychologist or a family counselor—such families can learn how to communicate.

But in a situation where the family is more open to the expression of feelings, a good way to overcome any reticence on the part of a child to talk about his or her feelings is, as I said earlier, to talk about your own. The child will quickly see that Mom and Dad have their own disappointments and deduce that "If it's all right for them to talk about it, then it's all right for me to talk to them about my concerns and problems." If the parent sets the example, the child will follow.

Then the ground will be set for a dialogue about the child's feelings about a career in sports. Remember that the questions you must ask aren't complex or profound, so don't make them more difficult by ruminating over them or by planning them in advance.

Don't forget the siblings. This advice doesn't just apply to the child involved in the decision. The rest of the children in the family have feelings about the possible sports career too, and they must be considered. So, for example, when you ask five-year-old Jane how she feels about what is going on with Jimmy and his baseball, you have to listen closely when she says, "I think it's fine, but will I still be able to have ice skating lessons?" This may sound like she's saying "yes" but it isn't a simple "yes," it's more of an expression of genuine anxiety. What she means is that whatever Jimmy does is all right with her if you can assure her that she won't be short-changed in the process or be loved any the less because Jimmy is going to be the star of the family for a while.

△ Balancing Desire and Ability △

Desire and ability are the central factors in a decision about whether or not a child should pursue a career in sports. The decision cannot be made on the basis of the youngster's desire while disregarding his athletic ability. Nor can it be made solely on the youngster's ability while disregarding his desire. A decision made on either of these bases alone could lead to failure. No, a parent must consider both factors and the youngster must consider them both as well.

This requires that all the parties involved step far enough away from the situation to objectively evaluate ability on the one hand and desire on the other, and to weigh them carefully.

△ Judging the Cost △

There are other considerations as well. One of these is the price to be paid. I'm not talking only of the financial price, which will likely be substantial, but the price that must be paid on the emotional scale, and the price that must be paid in sheer time. These prices are all high—in fact, they will more than likely result in a "sacrifice" on the part of everyone in the family, though the parents will bear the brunt.

These prices or commitments mean much more than simply carting the players back and forth to Little League once a week. Though success used to be predicated on simply "playing a lot of ball," in today's world the commitment to a sports career means special camps, special instruction year around, and special financial arrangements. The other children will have access to these advantages and yours will be at a disadvantage if he or she doesn't get the same kind of special care and attention. It all boils down to a simple equation: If two children with roughly the same natural physical ability are in competition, the one with the professional training—for example, attending a hitting school where a boy can be tutored in the mechanics of hitting as well as the basics—will almost always win the place on the team.

So, with this type of commitment on the horizon, it's absolutely imperative that parents sit down with their child and make certain that he or she understands what's really required of him. I've heard it scores of times, so I know that the child will undoubtedly say, "Yeah, folks, I'm ready for the sacrifices." All this means is that the child is living in the fantasy of being a professional, of the end product, and parents do the same thing. It's not that the youngster would refuse to go ahead if he knew the real requirements, but that he doesn't actually know what's going to be expected of him or the demands that it will put on his parents. The entire situation needs to be talked over at length with as many family members involved as possible. It's a considerably more complicated proposition than it appears on the surface. It's a romantic possibility but the reality is different because it includes not only athletic aspects but nonathletic aspects as well, such as establishing and maintaining a social life, attending school and making good grades, abiding by school schedules, and keeping a sleeping schedule. The youngster doesn't know what he's getting in to and parents play a crucial role in ushering the child through this period.

Training camps are an important element. They are expensive—as much as $5,000 a month—and the commitment must be kept. You don't send a child to these camps just because they offer a great experience, because they don't. Camps are hard work and not a wonderful experience that you, as a responsible parent, should expose your child to on a whim. Though I have to admit that trying it once will be a big help to a family and an athlete in deciding whether to continue on the professional path or to drop out.

The emotional investment is another matter, and it's different for the parent and the child. I've found that parents have the tendency to get their hopes up higher than the child—too high, in fact. Just as all students who go to Harvard don't come home lawyers, all athletes who go to football camp don't come home as Joe Namath. Parents can suffer more severely because they put all their hopes into the child's success. They are often naive about such camps.

The fact is, the emotional cost is almost always much higher than the financial cost, and unless the parent has examined his own feelings and motivations, and as a consequence of this exploration he is prepared for the possibility of the child's failure, the option should not be offered.

In reality, the child can't know the cost of the commitment to a sports career until he is advised and counseled, or gets to observe it or actually experiences it firsthand. And no matter how much counseling and preparation is done, neither the child or the parent will know what it's really like until the experience begins.

△ Judging the Necessary Commitment △

It is important to reiterate here that finances are just one part of the parents' responsibility. You must also assume the extra responsibilities of:

▷ Helping your child with school, since practice will take a good portion of each day and he won't have the same time available for doing his homework.

▷ Making sure that there is a balance in his or her social life.

▷ Providing encouragement, support, and advice during the up times and the down times.

▷ Helping develop all the other aspects of life that can easily be overlooked when the focus is so narrow.

The commitment of both parents here is the same as it would be with any gifted child. Athletic skill is a gift like the ability to play a musical instrument exceptionally well or the ability to do math at the highest levels. Studies of gifted children have shown that they don't develop their special potential unless they have a gifted parent—and by that I mean a parent who is prepared, for whatever reasons, to commit extraordinary effort to shepherding that child through the process that is necessary to develop that potential.

Moreover, it's simply not enough to excel in one area, be it math, or music, or sports. Being a well-rounded human being is also important, and the parents must be exceptional here as well.

Don't neglect the siblings. They are also part of the parents' commitment. Parents need to be sensitive to the rest of the children in the family. One of the requirements of having a serious athlete as a child is the support of the other children in equal measure in whatever it is they do. You can't have one child become successful and pay the price of having another child become neglected, troubled, depressed, or neurotic. Unless you can honestly tell yourself that you can provide your gifted child with everything he or she needs and *at the same time* provide other siblings with what they need—to feel loved, to feel important, to feel valued, to feel supported—you are making a mistake in committing yourself to the gifted child. Doing both takes more than a casual approach to parenting—it takes super parenting.

△ Judging the Rewards △

There are real rewards for parent and child in pursuing a sports career. Obviously, the major reward is the career itself, which offers the opportunity for recognition and financial gain. It's a way of life that offers the opportunity to develop self-esteem and have the pleasure of doing something excellently.

Success in sports in our society today is a unique situation. Because of the role sports play in our culture, there are very few successful athletes who are unsuccessful after their careers are over. Given the public perception of professional sports and the adoration given to pro athletes, if a person gets the opportunity to perform on the pro level, even the lowest rung, it carries tremendous reward which can be used in every aspect of life.

The opportunity to be a professional puts a person in a category that is quite a bit above the average. It opens career doors for even the marginal professional athlete. That person can toss his resume on the desk and it will get a different kind of attention than someone with equal ability and experience. All other things being equal, the pro experience can be parlayed into opportunities that a nonathlete can't get.

It is important to point out however that the rewards of a successful career may not be all that the athlete has imagined. Public recognition and adulation may preclude his having the privacy to enjoy himself and his wealth. Nor will his wealth and talent necessarily make his life easy. Often an athlete feels that all he needs to do is go out and play and all other life problems will be resolved. He believes that he is immune from tragedy, divorce, sickness, even death. In rare instances this may be the case, but for the most part it is not.

△ Emphasize the Process, Not the Outcome △

One final point. In modern American society, there is the sentiment that if we don't win, or don't get some material gain at the end of a pursuit, the thing that we did was a waste of time and effort. So many times my clients talk about "wasted effort" and what they really mean is that if they did something and it was not "successful," it wasn't worth doing. That is a rather absurd concept. We don't do things only because of how they are going to come out. We do them because we enjoy the doing of them and we get something out of the doing.

This concept applies particularly to the parent and the athletic child. If you as a parent can enjoy the process of helping your child, in whatever way you can, to maximize his or her athletic (or any other) potential, then the outcome becomes secondary. Even if things don't go as planned, you won't feel like you've failed in the end because you've enjoyed doing it. The plus factors for parents are enormous: You're spending more time with your child; you're sharing new things; and you're learning things about yourself as a human being and a parent. If you approach it this way, you can't lose. You will have established a foundation for your relationship with your child that will last a lifetime. This is the product. Your child's athletic success is the by-product. If you maintain this emphasis, everyone involved will be in good shape.

If you can adopt this perspective in all the spheres of parenting, then by your example you can help your child adopt this approach to life as well. And if the child comes to value the process of doing something above the outcome, he is going to be a much happier human being and later on in life he in turn will be a much happier parent.

CHAPTER

9

△ △

The Recreational Path

*T*ODAY'S PROFESSIONAL ATHLETES bear about as much resemblance to Pete Rose or Arnold Palmer as the Wright brothers plane does to the Space Shuttle.

As recently as twenty years ago an athlete could become a professional in most sports virtually without specialized training, private coaching, or a major financial investment by his parents. Baseball stars like Rose almost always got their coaching from their fathers and their playing experience in their home towns in leagues that were sponsored by local merchants. Palmer learned to play golf from his father and honed his skills on a public golf course. Because of this, there was little difference in the way youngsters approached their favorite game. Whether they had professional aspirations or just wanted to play ball with their buddies, they just went out and played.

This isn't possible today. High salaries and international recognition have changed the world of sports to the degree that if a child and his parents want to follow the professional path they must approach the training process (the training *years*, in reality) with a combination of business acumen, perseverance, and sensitivity that is frequently hard to manage.

△

In other words, just sending Susie to the neighborhood gymnastics class will not be enough to produce a champion, even a city champion. She may learn some movements and even be good at what she does, but she simply won't be professional enough. Similarly, letting Frankie play third base for the local Little League team isn't going to help him get into the big leagues or even to win a baseball scholarship to college. In both cases—in fact, in all cases—highly skilled professionals are now produced by highly skilled professionals. A professional career is only for the strong-willed, the exceptionally talented, and those willing and able to spend the money to get the desired results.

With this in mind, let me take a moment to distinguish once again between the requirements of the professional path and those of the recreational path in American sports in the 1980s. The professional path has these specific characteristics:

▷ It's a job

▷ Special training camps are a must

▷ The young athlete in training will most likely live and train away from home

▷ Private coaching is a must

▷ Private tutors will be needed to maintain the youngster's academic standing

▷ The best performance comes from using the best, and therefore the most expensive, equipment

▷ The young athlete must play against the best competition

▷ The psychological and physical pressures are heavy

▷ There is a considerable financial investment required

▷ There is a huge emotional investment on the part of both parents and athlete

▷ The entire family is involved

▷ Total dedication to the task is essential

▷ There is every reason to believe that if the athlete is successful there will eventually be a return on the financial investment in the form of salary and fees for endorsements and personal appearances

If you chose this path, you have to accept the fact that all of the above are part of the package.

Until fifteen years ago or so it was possible for a talented athlete to become a top amateur in his or her sport and then go on to become a tennis, golf, or gymnastics instructor if they didn't have the ability or the desire to become a full-time professional. This too has changed. With the advent of open sports events, the dedicated amateur athlete has all but disappeared from the American sports scene. This means the youngster who "only" wants to be an Olympic performer or a teaching professional must follow the same course (with all the requirements listed above) as the youngster training for a competitive professional career.

Taking the recreational path, on the other hand, is not like taking a job, though the time and effort involved may still produce a return on investment in the form of a college scholarship or some other kind of official recognition like medals and trophies. But, unlike the professional path, the recreational path has several possible variations:

1. Serious participation at the interscholastic level;

2. Serious participation at the college level;

3. Intramural and other organized competition;

4. Casual participation for diversion, health, fitness, and fun;

5. High-level amateur play, which by virtue of the time involved is more often the preserve of the wealthy.

Serious interscholastic competition requires a certain dedication on the part of the young athlete, but it doesn't require an absolute commitment to the long-term goal of becoming a professional. Possibly what distinguishes this level of competition is that it usually has the elements of fun and the joy of competition—that is, it doesn't have the deadly serious aspects of professional sports training, where the fun has been wrung out of the process. In fact, many talented youngsters who never compete in organized sports in high school go on to college and are able to make the school team in a given sport. This testifies to the fact that, at this level, a childhood dedicated to preparation for serious preparation isn't necessary to compete successfully.

Similarly, an athlete who competes in varsity sports at the college level doesn't need quite the same degree of training or dedication as the athlete who has chosen the professional path. The number of athletic scholarships available at the major colleges is limited and those scholarships go to the exceptionally talented. The chances of the good, natural athlete becoming a scholarship player are slim, but the chances of the natural athlete playing college-level sports are not bad. And surprisingly in this day and age many college athletes, especially those who play at universities where sports are de-emphasized, participate for the fun of it.

Intramural sports and organized sports teams in industrial and business leagues are good alternatives for the competitive but less dedicated athlete. Playing softball, volleyball, basketball, touch football, and other sports for the thrill of competition and the socialization is a rewarding way to stay physically and mentally fit.

Of course, there are many more athletes who run or play tennis and golf and other sports just for fitness, fun, and social reasons. This variation on the recreational path is where most of us eventually find ourselves, even those of us who fancy ourselves to be good athletes.

On the high-amateur level, the best athletes are often the privileged few who can devote their efforts (not their spare time) to a particular sport or sports. These people can often compete with professionals but they don't make their living from sports and the reasons they pursue their pastime so seriously are as varied as the athletes themselves.

△ Dealing with the Decision Not to Go Professional △

For the athlete who has had professional aspirations but for any number of reasons has chosen the recreational path, the pressure is now truly off. There may be some residue of doubt about the decision, some second thoughts in the minds of both parents and children, but if all the facets of the question have been carefully considered, then the family and the athlete will soon rest easy knowing that the right, the realistic, and the informed decision was reached.

If, until now, your youngster had seriously been headed down the professional path, this will be a somewhat rocky period and your continued involvement is important. Here are some ways you can help:

1. Be available to discuss the decision with your youngster as often as he or she wants to talk about it.

2. Emphasize the real reasons for the decision: for example, don't say that the reason is the cost of training when it is really a lack of talent.

3. Continue to encourage your child to participate in athletics and continue to play with him or her.

4. Make sure the message is clear that even though your child isn't going to be a star, he is still a star to you.

An important point to note here is that the decision to follow the recreational path doesn't preclude any and all sports competition for your youngster; it only changes the focus of that competition. True, you won't be sending him or her to an expensive tennis camp that emphasizes training for a career in tennis and caters only to the cream of the country's young players. But if your youngster still wants to go to a tennis camp or take private lessons, there are plenty of places and coaches that stress the development of technique and skills while deemphasizing the "win at all costs" aspects of competition that are necessary emotional components of the professional's psyche. In fact, there are many more of these kinds of camps and coaches than there are of the professional type.

Let me use my own personal experience to illustrate what I mean here. At age thirteen, I thought I was on my way to a professional career in either baseball or football. I was a first team player in both sports at my high school and was considered a good prospect for a college scholarship, especially in baseball. Then, at some point during my junior year, I realized that there was more to life than locker rooms and liniment, and I decided, with the help of my parents, to direct more of my energies to my school work, to developing a social life outside of my limited circle of athlete friends, and to begin to look at college as more than a four-year stop on the way to life as a professional athlete.

After the decision was made, I felt relieved in many ways because I didn't have to fulfill my own and my parent's expectations, but I was also sad for a time because I had spent a good part of my developing years moving toward a goal and now that goal had been removed. For a while I vacillated between the emotions of grief at giving up my idea and elation for having done so. I went through a period where my mood changed from day to day. Some days I was pleased with myself and my parents and some days I was mad at them and myself for the choice we had all made. I also had to contend with my former teammates, who couldn't understand my decision. Even though I was still playing on the baseball team, and playing well, I was no longer the same part of the team as I'd been before and much less a part of the locker-room scene.

I also had to deal with that feeling athletes have that we are somehow better than nonathletes, that we're made of stronger stuff and therefore superior in some undefined way. This sense of importance is a combination of factors that include:

▷ The knowledge that you are in control of your body;

▷ The knowledge that you have specific talents that few people have;

▷ The adulation of your peers who are not athletes;

▷ The approval of your parents;

▷ The approval of coaches;

▷ Recognition in the community.

I could immediately sense the loss of some of these elements that so bolster a teenager's self-esteem, but there was nothing I could do about the loss but to accept it and move on. I had an uneasy feeling for several months that made me wonder almost daily if I'd done the right thing.

But my parents were completely supportive and when I began to make some new friends outside of sports, my anxiety about the decision began to fade. As I began to take part in non-sports activities—going to movies, eating what I wanted, talking about subjects other than sports—I relaxed even more. And in the nonsports world, the place where most people live, I quickly began to lose that jock mentality about being superior. In less than six months, I did an about-face. I was now looking at athletes as if they were the inferior ones and I began to feel that I'd managed to escape just in time.

That was more than thirty years ago now. I have never regretted my decision, but there are still times when I fantasize about what might have been or feel a twinge of envy when I watch a great athlete perform. When I come back to reality, however, it's clear to me that the course I took was the right one for me.

This is easy enough for me to say, as a mature adult looking at the past, but you, as a parent, will have to take the responsibility for helping your child over these same rough spots after your decision has been made. That help and support may be necessary for some time. This is especially true if a professional sports career was considered a truly obtainable goal by your youngster and by you. You will have to work on your own responses as well, because parents are usually as deeply involved and committed to this dream as the child—sometimes more so.

When I think about my own situation, I now understand that my parents were going through some of the same withdrawal symptoms as I was, only being adults they were able to see the big picture in a way that I couldn't.

Over the years, I've worked with many parents who have suffered through this period of disorientation and frustration with their youngsters who are good, but not professional-caliber, athletes. Through these conversations with parents and their youngsters I've developed guidelines which parents have found helpful in their discussions about the subject with their children. Essentially, these guidelines point out that though it may not seem that way, the fact is, the youngster who chooses the recreational path has many possibilities open to him or her. These include:

1. The opportunity to pursue an active athletic life in a variety of sports;

2. The chance to develop skills with the accent on fun;

3. The opportunity to play without worrying about winning;

4. Emphasizing participation;

5. The development of skills that will be useful later in life for both pleasure and business.

The death of a dream is always difficult to deal with psychologically. It makes no difference if that dream is to become an athlete, an actor, or a scientist. Parents must help their children through this period of mourning and when this is done with sensitivity, the child that comes out on the other side will be psychologically healthy.

As I've said many times throughout this book, I feel athletics are an important element in the life of a child and of an adult. I also feel that, except for a few exceptionally stable athletes, the recreational path is the better way to go.

10

△   △

The Professional Path

Note: This chapter may not be for everyone. If you and your child have opted for the recreational path described in the previous chapter, much of the discussion in this chapter will not be directly relevant. That said, we are still dealing with parent-child interaction, and for that reason I think this section is important for all parents.

WITH SOME EXCEPTIONS, the preparation for a career in professional sports doesn't need to begin until the age of twelve or thirteen. That's the time when the entire family must decide to make the commitments that will turn Jennie into an Olympic diver and Bobby into a major league pitcher.

At first glance this may appear to be a five- or ten-year commitment at most, but the reality is that, like all the commitments you make when you have a child, it is long term. Guiding your son or daughter into and through an athletic career is more like a twenty-year commitment because your child's professional career, once it's established, will still be a source of pleasure and sometimes of pain for you.

This parental commitment to a professional athlete career for a child actually breaks down into three stages. Stage One starts when the child begins a serious training program, at about age eighteen. Stage Two continues until the youngster enters college or when he goes to the Olympics or begins to get paid for what he does. Stage Three continues throughout the athlete's professional career and in some cases for the rest of the athlete's life.

△

Parental involvement is greatest during Stage One, less critical but still important in Stage Two, and peripheral in Stage Three because so much is out of their control. In this third stage, however, the parent's emotional involvement is just as high if not higher than ever because this is the period when all the years of hard work begin to bear fruit.

△ The Parents' Role in Stage One △

In Stage One there are many things the committed family must consider. These include:

1. Selecting a coach

2. Overseeing the young athlete's training

3. Helping the youngster adjust socially, psychologically, physically, and academically

4. Preserving the family unit

5. Helping the athlete during the off-season

6. Helping the athlete deal with injuries and interim failures

7. Planning alternatives and options

Selecting a Coach

I've mentioned several times that the choice of the right coach, the right training camp, or a combination of the two, is critical for the young athlete who, with his parents, has chosen the professional path. In fact, it is the most important decision to be made. This is primarily because, given today's competition, success is virtually impossible without superior coaching. Good coaches are in business for three reasons: to produce quality athletes, to build a reputation for themselves as coaches of champions, and to make money, but not necessarily in that order.

Unfortunately, a few coaches, even some of those who are highly thought of, are more concerned with their own reputations than with any of the other factors involved in the coaching of young people. The worst of these are insecure martinets and egotists who are in the business primarily because their position gives them control over other people's lives and for the money.

Thankfully, the majority of the men and women who are professional coaches are dedicated not only to excellence but to the well-being of the student, not just as an athlete but as a whole person.

The choice of the right coach is not unlike the choice of a family doctor, and you should make the choice by using some of the same criteria. When you shop for a doctor you look for a person with the right credentials—the right education, experience, and technical skills necessary to treat you—and a bedside manner that makes you feel comfortable. The same is true of coaches. Your choice for a first coach for your child must have the experience and technical skills you're looking for. Just as you wouldn't use a brain surgeon if you have a sore muscle, you wouldn't select someone who works best polishing the skills of established professionals for a child who is just beginning.

In the beginning stages, you need someone who understands more about the fundamentals than about the fine points of the sport. In short, you're looking for someone to teach the sport in depth.

But credentials are only part of the story. The coach's personal approach—his bedside manner—must be sympathetic. He must be sensitive to the tender feelings of both youngsters and their parents. You are establishing what may be a long-term relationship, and as in any such relationship both parties should be as compatible as possible. Because there is so much at stake and so many things can go wrong, you will have to be able to communicate back and forth in order to ensure progress. And keep in mind that, like a doctor, you may want to change coaches in the future without rancor or recriminations. In fact, it's possible that you will use several coaches during your child's progressive developmental stages.

You also know that there is usually more than one good doctor or medical specialist that is right for you or your case. The same is true with coaches. There is rarely only one potential coach for your child. Many coaches like to think they are the sole source of knowlege and experience in a given sport, just as doctors do, but there is a pool of general and specific knowledge about each sport and most coaches share this knowledge. There are many equally qualified man and woman in each field, so don't hesitate to interview three or four or more potential people.

Certainly, some coaches are better than others and occasionally there is someone who is considered "the top man in the field." This may be the person you want to seek out at some time in your child's training, but remember that the second facet of good coaching is the ability to communicate. If the "top man" is brusque, authoritarian, and rude—in short, if he has a lousy bedside manner—then he isn't worth the trouble he will cause for you and your young athlete. Coaches must be carefully matched to the temperament and the talents of your youngster. Don't be susceptible to the dynamic of "authority," an aura that some coaches project either consciously or unconsciously, which often seduces parents into making the wrong choice. You wouldn't go to a doctor if you didn't like him personally and this is true of coaches as well.

As a starting point, try to determine your needs and your youngster's needs, both for technical training and for emotional support. Here are some questions to ask yourself about any coach or training program you may be considering:

1. Do you need a private coach, a camp with a highly regarded coach, or a combination of the two?

2. Does the coach seem to be interested in you and your youngster as people as well as clients?

3. Does he or she seem rigid and inflexible, or sensitive and flexible?

4. Does his or her approach allow for individual differences in talents and personalities?

5. Does the program include a "normal" academic program, or does it require the use of private tutors?

6. Is it a live-in program?

7. Does the program allow for family input and participation, or are you supposed to turn your child over to the coach?

8. Does the coach make periodic evaluations of progress to the parents?

9. Does the coach use positive reinforcement techniques, or negative and punitive methods?

10. Does he or she set realistic goals?

11. Do assistants do most of the real coaching?

12. Does the regimen allow for socialization with nonprogram participants?

13. Is there a sports psychologist on staff?

14. Is the program within your budget?

15. Would you like to be a student with this coach yourself?

Obviously, it isn't necessary for a coach or a camp to meet all of these requirements to the letter, but it is important that you get answers to these questions before putting your money into a contract (yes, many coaches and camps require contracts) that will bind you to any program.

In order to answer these questions meaningfully you must, as I've said, know your child's needs and his personality. You must know if he responds better in a highly structured situation or in one where there is more permissiveness, whether he needs special treatment or not, whether he needs constant support or whether he's independent and achieves on his own.

Since the choice of a coach or a camp program is one of the most important and difficult decisions you'll have to make along the professional path, let's examine each of the questions above in more detail.

1. Frankly, it's hard to know if your child needs private coaching, a camp atmosphere, or both. But in my experience working with parents and their youngsters, I've found that combining the two is often the answer. First, I think it's psychologically more sound for the young athlete to live at home during the school year and this means private coaching before and after school and on weekends. This gives the youngster the chance to grow up in a normal atmosphere instead of being sent to the equivalent of a boarding school that teaches nothing but sports. This arrangement is better academically and emotionally, and it's also less expensive.

In the first two or three years of the training program, a summer sports camp is a good supplement to the young athlete's daily routine because it offers the child a chance to get away from the pressures of the private coaching sessions and the added pressures that are inevitable in the home. It also gives him a chance to interact with his peers, which is usually not possible on a home schedule that demands practicing at 6:30 a.m. and 4:30 p.m., spending some time with the family, and doing homework.

2. You want a coach who treats parents and young athletes as human beings rather than clients. What you are forming is more of a partnership than a client-customer relationship, and you need to make your feelings known about this. Your initial meeting with the coach will give you an idea of the way he operates, but you should make it a point to observe the coach in action on several occasions. You'll also want to observe how the coach interacts with his staff and with the students in the program.

3. These meetings will also give you the opportunity to make a judgment about the coach's level of sensitivity and flexibility. A sense of humor is often a good indicator of a person's sensitive nature, but the best way to determine his feelings and the rigidity of his approach is close observation of his reactions to your questions about the structure of the program. If he is defensive and evasive, or if he says things like, "This is the only way we do it here," you may be in the wrong place.

4. No two athletes are alike, so no single approach is right in a coaching program. For example, the attempt to mold a youngster's tennis stroke to a specific pattern will not work in many cases because bodies are different in size, weight, flexibility, strength, and coordination. Personalities are also different and the psychology that works with one athlete may not work at all with another.

5. Private coaches usually hold their training sessions before and after regular school hours and on weekends. These instructors are not directly responsible for an athlete's academic progress, but it should be one of their considerations. In many cases, however, these teachers place academics far down on the list of priorities. Still, when the training takes place at home, it is the parents' responsibility to make sure school work gets down correctly and on time.

If you choose to send your child to a full-time training program away from home, you should select one that includes a normal academic program—that is, one with an arrangement for a regular day school. If tutoring is added to the regular school program, it can be helpful in providing your child with the extra assistance he needs to meets the heavy demands of school and training program. But tutoring should only be remedial and supplemental, never a substitute for the regular school environment. A training program that offers only tutors is not the place you want to put your child.

6. If you choose a live-in program, you will want to know not only about schooling but about visiting schedules, holidays, and summer vacations. Some camps discourage visits by parents and others welcome them. Some camps allow for extended holidays and vacations and others require almost constant attendance year-round. There is nothing inherently right or wrong with either schedule as long as the decision for one or the other is made mutually by parents and athlete. But be aware that both kinds of plans are available.

7. Some coaches demand that parents turn their child over to them, much like some boarding schools do. The coach may give the following rationale for this: "I can't possibly turn a child into a world-class athlete if I have parents interfering with my methods." I believe that this approach is questionable and I feel the same way about a regular boarding school. A training program should not be a boot camp that isolates trainees from family and friends. A good program will present many opportunities for parental input and participation and this in turn allows parents to continually assess the coach's approach and the progress of their child. The point is, the youngster is *your* child and *your* ultimate responsibility. It isn't good parenting to turn that responsibility over to someone else, either at a sports camp or at a boarding school.

8. Any coach worth his reputation will make periodic reports to parents about the progress of the child. In most cases, there is no reason to doubt the validity of these evaluations, but coaches have been known to make unrealistic evaluations. There are coaches who will provide parents with glowing reports even when their child is not doing particularly well in a program. Some coaches do this to keep parents at bay and keep youngsters in the program. Others will be more modest in their appraisals but not indicate that there are problems. If a child is not making fast progress but still shows potential that is one thing, but if the potential isn't there—after a fair trial—then parents and the athlete are entitled to know. The good coaches will tell you the truth as soon as they know it.

9. There are many ways of teaching, but the punitive method is not the one I recommend. For a variety of reasons—insecurity, frustration, the mistaken idea that louder is more authoritative— many coaches berate their students at top volume, thinking they will get a better response through this method than they would through encouraging and cajoling. Many youngsters become frightened and anxious under this kind of treatment and perform even more poorly than before because of the coach's behavior. Coaches should observe, criticize, and correct. Criticism is a necessary ingredient in teaching and coaching, and the carrot and stick approach will work in many cases, but the stick—the criticism—doesn't have to be applied at a full yell to be effective. From a psychological point of view, I know this method doesn't work. The fragile psyche of a young athlete reacts better to honey than vinegar. A coach's mannerisms will give him away, and you should be able to tell almost immediately if the man is a tyrant or a benevolent dictator.

10. Realistic goals are crucial in any activity. If a coach tells you that he will make a professional golfer out of your daughter in two years, he's not telling the truth. Certainly, goals have to be flexible, because development problems and injuries can slow progress, but there is no way a coach can determine how long it will take to turn a raw talent into a polished performer who is able to compete with the best in the world. Don't be afraid to ask a coach to set goals, but make it clear that you expect those goals to be achievable and the length of time allowed for substantial progress to be within the realm of possibility.

11. In many sports camps it is the assistants that do most of the real teaching. This isn't necessarily bad, because they are usually younger than the camp director and relate more closely to the students. They are also professionals or former professionals, so their skills are not in question. What is in question is whether you are paying for the coaching skills of the director or for those of his assistants. Make sure that you find out in advance who will be doing the actual instruction and evaluation. And be sure to talk at some length with this person and to give your child a chance to meet him or her as well. You don't want to pay for something you aren't getting.

12. Many training programs, whether with private coaches or in camps, simply don't allow enough time for socialization,

especially time to mix with youngsters who are not in the program. Concentration on training is necessary, but it isn't necessary to spend every waking moment playing or talking about playing. There are precious few social opportunities for a child in professional training, so programs that make an effort to provide those chances are worthy of your attention.

Let me point out one more time that the career path is the job path, and children in training to be professional athletes are abnormal. They aren't "sick," obviously, but it isn't normal for a youngster to be thrust into a career long before the normal time for that choice and especially into a program that essentially deprives a child of his or her chance to be child. Therefore, seize every opportunity to let your youngster interact with "regular" children his or her own age.

13. I don't know many professional sports camps that have a sports psychologist on staff, but I think such a person is invaluable. I think the reason they don't have them is that most coaches think they are psychologists. Believe me, they aren't. Psychologists aren't coaches either, but the combination of the two professional skills can save a lot of young psyches from serious harm. If you're looking at a camp with a psychologist on staff, give that camp extra consideration.

14. As an adult, I've always felt that a good rule of thumb for judging a sports camp or a private coach was whether I would like to be a participant in that program. There are some people who create an atmosphere of quiet authority and leadership that makes you say to yourself that you, as an adult, would like to work with this man. If you can find that situation, I strongly recommend that you take it.

Answering the above questions for yourself is not all that is involved in selecting a coach. The decision must be made in cooperation with your child. And it isn't enough to simply ask your child, "Do you like this man?" or "Do you like this camp?" You have to elicit some real opinions here with questions like:

▷ What people do you like here?

▷ What people don't you like?

▷ What did you like about the other kids? What didn't you like about them?

▷ What did you like about the room where you'd be staying? What didn't you like about it?

▷ What did you like about the food?

▷ What did you like about the camp director?

▷ What did you like about the coach you'll be working with? What didn't you like about him?

▷ Would you like to spend the summer (or winter) here?

Though the youngster is not making the choice himself—that is the parent's responsibility—he should participate in the decision and feel that he is participating. The answers to these kinds of questions should give you a good idea of his or her feelings on the matter.

Overseeing the Athlete's Training

Once the coaching decision has been made, the athlete and his parents must focus on making the situation work. From the child's point of view, this means working hard and fulfilling his or her end of the long-term bargain made with the parents and coach.

And the parents have more to do than just pay the bills; much more. You only have to look at the headlines on the sports pages to see some of the problems today's athletes are experiencing. As a psychologist I see the majority of these problems—from drug use, to betting, to rape and other criminal acts—as the result of retarded social development brought on by the isolation of the athlete from real life situations that require actual decision-making and interaction with regular people.

In my opinion, this is a direct result of the special care and attention an athlete receives from his parents, coaches, friends, teachers, and the public. This attention tells the youngster, as early as age thirteen or fourteen, that he is somehow better than his peers and that he is worthy of treatment not afforded to others. This sort of attention can't help but inflate a young person's ego and make him think he is above it all, including the law.

This myth is further perpetuated by college programs that offer athletes private dormitories, training table meals, meaningless classes, fancy cars, money, no-show jobs and even the sexual favors of women. And since athletes usually socialize with other athletes they tend to feed each other's egos until they feel they can buy and use drugs, drive drunk, and commit other crimes with impunity. We've seen the results of this superman attitude on the police blotter and the obituary page.

Of course, criminal behavior and drug overdoses are the exception. The more common distortions of the athlete's life include the following examples taken from my own practice:

▷ The nineteen-year-old gymnast who couldn't add, subtract, or handle money because she spent so little time in school during her years of training

▷ The college basketball star who couldn't read a book, a newspaper, or even a driver's license application because he was given a free ride through elementary and high school and then through college

▷ The eleven-year-old equestrian who was unable to talk to strangers without bursting into tears because she had never been exposed to people who weren't involved in her sport

▷ The high school football player who has almost daily fights with his older brother in order to prove that he is an athlete with "special" powers

▷ The nine-year-old swimmer who ran away from swimming camp in the middle of the night because he wasn't able to swim lap times that pleased his coach

▷ The eighteen-year-old tennis player who broke his three best racquets and refused to attend another class because he and his parents had set unrealistic goals for his progress

Some of these reactions relate to burnout, a very real psychological (and sometimes physical) response to years of heavy and continuous training. It has happened to many great athletes in every sport, but it happens more often in the individual sports like tennis, swimming, skating, skiing, and gymnastics. It happens less often in team sports because most team sports are seasonal and give the athlete time to rest, relax, play other sports, and get out from under the pressure for a few months.

But burnout isn't the whole story. Young people and adults react differently to the demands of sports training just as they do to everyday pressures like those of school or the business world. The symptoms of these reactions can take the form of heavy drinking, chain smoking, drug use, erratic eating and sleeping habits, headaches and other psycho-physical ailments, temper tantrums, and other forms of self-destructive and antisocial behavior. There is no protection against these problems except that knowing about them in advance makes their onset, should it occur, a slightly less traumatic experience.

Again, I am not giving these examples to frighten parents of young athletes, only to warn you that at some point your child may well react negatively to the constant pressures of training, competition, and performance. Through experience adults are better prepared to handle the vicissitudes of life. Young people have no such experience and often can't cope with the need to satisfy their own needs and those of all the adults around them.

Fortunately, along with this warning, I can offer some suggestions on how to prevent, or at least mitigate, these unhappy developments. Because as parents you are ultimately responsible for your child's well-being, you should consciously work to create a balance in your young athlete's life, a balance that will make him or her a more well-rounded person. It's obvious that by virtue of taking the professional path, his sport is going to be the most important element in your child's life, so part of your job is to see that the other aspects of life are attended to as well.

Schooling

Academics are important. If the athlete is living at home he or she should be in a regular school program. School is an integrative and communal experience. A youngster learns more than facts in school. It is a place for social development as well. Outside of school, be sure that time is set aside for study, that homework is done, that help with school work is given as needed, that tutors are engaged if necessary, that teachers are contacted regularly for progress reports, and that any problems are discussed with your child as soon as they arise.

If the child is living away from home, you won't be able to make these arrangements yourself, but you still have the responsibility to check on academic progress and to suggest alternatives and rememdies. Again, tutoring can be helpful when there are specific problems, but it should only be remedial and supplemental, never a substitute for the regular school environment.

When a youngster reaches college age, he or she should take advantage of the opportunities college offers for education and socialization. The top-flight athlete has a distinct advantage over the nonathlete in that he or she will more than likely be offered scholarships to several institutions. I advise parents to urge their children to attend college if they are qualified, because a college education is an insurance policy against that time when professional sports careers end (and this sometimes occurs suddenly) because of deteriorating skills, age, or injury.

Social Life

There *is* a life outside of sports. The whole world does not turn on sports nor is everyone interested in the outcome of last night's game, the size of a person's biceps, or the type of diet an athlete eats. For this reason, the parents of a young athlete in training should make every effort to see that their son or daughter has a social life that is separate from the group they train with. I once had a young figure skater as a patient who was severely depressed because she had no friends at all. She skated with her coach before school, then went to classes at a regular high school where she was often too tired to pay attention to the other students. After school, she skated again with her coach, then went home, had dinner, did her homework, and went to bed. She saw other boys and girls in school but she knew she didn't have the time to socialize after school so she never made friends.

A regular social environment for the athlete is important for two reasons, one immediate and the other long term. The immediate reason is that all youngsters need exposure to, and the stimulation of, a variety of young people with different ideas, backgrounds, and interests. The constant companionship of other athletes can create a youngster who feels elite but who is at the same time withdrawn because of an inability to relate to the rest of the world. The long-term reason for expanding a youngster's social horizons is that the post-sports career world is not made up just of former athletes. Later business and social contacts will more likely be nonsports-oriented.

Family Life

Your career-path athlete is going to receive your special attention, of that there can be no doubt. But if there are siblings, those youngsters should receive the same attention afforded the athlete and be offered opportunities to take part in activities of equal value. If all a family's resources, both emotional and financial, are used in meeting the athletic child's needs, the siblings will eventually suffer emotionally and the entire family structure will be threatened.

Moreover, make sure you incorporate your athletic child in the family as normally as possible. It should be made clear that after training, everything else is done like the rest of the members of the family do it.. He should perform regular household tasks like doing the dishes, mowing the lawn, and keeping his room in order. Everyone in a family has a different goal that fact must be recognized. The athletic child should be treated no better and no worse than his siblings.

Immaturity and Loss of Childhood

As I mentioned, the decision to become a professional athlete can't be taken lightly in today's world. Though we often have the tendency not to take sports seriously because they are after all only games, an athletic career is a job and must be approached like any other job.

The key difference between a sports career and a career in law, for example, is that most lawyers don't begin their careers until after college, at age twenty-two or twenty-three. Athletes must start their careers at age thirteen, a tender age in all ways and more tender still when the pressures of athletic performance are added to the normal pressures of being a teenager in a modern society.

What we're doing, therefore, is asking a child to undertake a task that is difficult for most mature adults—that is, to look and plan ahead and to devote all their time and effort to achieving a single goal. To do this, the young athlete must give up a major portion of his or her childhood, and both parents and the child must recognize this fact.

We expect the athlete to handle his life in an adult way, but the fact is, the young athlete is just that, young and still a child. A friend of mine who used to own a professional basketball franchise once told me that it was very hard for him to look at a seven-foot player, who physically had all the attributes of an adult, and realize that the person was often still only a teenager, not able to talk business or to talk about anything but sports, not able to negotiate a contract, not even able to have a legal drink at a bar. In other words, young athletes have all the physical attributes of adults, but in many ways they are still children.

In other ways, athletes are social misfits because they have never had the chance to be normal people. For that, and other reasons, it isn't the least uncommon for young athletes to grow bitter and resentful toward their parents because, a bit later in life, they feel they've been robbed of their chance to be a child and to fit in socially with their peer group. Of course, they are right, but the problem is difficult and after the fact, there is little parents can do about it.

There is probably no way to totally prevent this feeling of resentment, but it can be softened to a certain extent if both parent and child discuss the realities of the life everyone in the family is beginning before it begins. I can't give you the words to use, but it must be done, even if haltingly, because the consequences can be severe.

Injuries

All top athletes feel they are supermen who can't be injured, at least not seriously. There is abundant evidence to the contrary, but the athlete's mind (with good psychological reasons) doesn't permit the possibility of injury to enter his thought processes. If he did, the chances are he couldn't perform.

But it's clear that physical injuries do occur. They are a fact of athletic life regardless of the age of the athlete. Youngsters may have fewer serious injuries and broken bones than older competitors because they are less brittle and more relaxed, but they have them. And even the best conditioned body sometimes breaks down under the constant pounding of training and competition. Obviously, physical injuries can be very serious, but the physical problem of a pulled muscle or a twisted knee is often less painful than the impact the injury delivers to the psyche of the athlete. The physical injury tells the mind that the body is not impervious and in the final analysis, the psychological effects of a physcial injury can be more debilitating than the physical problem itself.

Since we know injuries can't be prevented, the best thing for the young athlete to do psychologically is to anticipate that at some time he or she will be injured, that in essence injuries go with the territory. I know this is easier said than done because

I've worked with athletes and I have had great difficulty in getting them to believe that the possibility of injury exists. Denial is the classic defense and athletes are masters at it.

Still, there is no denying that pushing the body to its limits can result in breakdowns of tissue, muscle, and bone so an athlete who is mentally prepared for that occurrence will suffer fewer psychological doubts about his ability to recover than the athlete who professes invulnerability and never admits to the possibility of injury.

The main element in this mental preparation is a firm commitment to keep training after the injury. It's important to recognize that there are few injuries that totally incapacitate an athlete. Yet many otherwise sensible people will stop training completely even when the injury doesn't prevent them from training in some other way.

Several years ago a professional football player was referred to me because he was concerned about his future and his ability to come back after an injury to a leg muscle. His injury was serious but not career-threatening. I quickly realized, however, that his attitude *was* career-threatening. As soon as he realized that his hamstring pull would keep him from running for several weeks, he became depressed. Instead of going to the gym and using weights to continue working on his upper body strength, he vegetated in front of the television set eating potato chips and feeling sorry for himself, and at the same time he let the rest of his body deteriorate. He also began to turn on his wife and his friends when they tried to console and encourage him.

Then, after three weeks of inactivity, he suddenly decided to test his leg. He realized that it was still quite tender but he went to a neighborhood track and started to run. In two minutes he had reinjured the hamstring even more severely. He told me that as he hobbled to his car he had tears in his eyes because he felt his leg would never recover. After that, his depression deepened.

I worked with this man for several weeks and we did make some progress. He started to go to the gym on a semiregular basis and he eventually recovered and returned to the team. But he was never able to regain his previous form, at least not in his mind.

This player's attitude was his major obstacle. He just couldn't come to grips with the reality of being injured. This was then compounded by the fact that for many weeks he refused to train because he was too confused, fearful, and embarrassed. His leg problem wouldn't have prevented him from using his upper body, but he let it prevent him from doing so. In the process, his overall physical condition broke down along with his attitude about training. His self-esteem suffered, his self-doubts intruded on his life, and his depression grew with each passing day. I was able to help him in some ways, but I couldn't convince him that his injury was temporary and I couldn't train for him, and that was the ultimate problem.

Studies have shown that exercise is an antidote to depression. In fact, vigorous exercise is now being used by therapists as treatment for severely depressed people who are not athletes. The results of these experiments indicate that the stimulation of physical movement has positive effects on brain chemistry which in turn lessens depression.

Thus, for the injured athlete, it is not only physically important but it is psychologically important to continue training because the exercise will fight depression. Moreover, since the routine of training has become a habit in his life, continuing to work out can lift the initial despair and despondency caused by the injury by helping him maintain his identity as an athlete and his self-esteem.

When injuries hit the young athlete the results are the same as they are for the mature athlete. Parents need to encourage, and if necessary demand, that their youngster continue to train. If the injury is to the upper body, then train the legs on a stationary bicycle or with weights. If it is to the hips, legs, ankles, or feet, continue to train the upper body with weights. In either case, swimming is recommended because it helps maintain aerobic fitness with less strain on the bones and muscles.

If there has been no mental preparation, even minor injuries can end careers. An understanding of the realities of the situation can keep this from happening.

The Off-Season

Varied off-season activities can prevent burnout. I have mentioned the phenomenon of burnout, but it needs further consideration because it can have the dramatic effect of suddenly ending an athletic career, usually a career that seems to be on the rise rather than in decline.

In essence, burnout occurs when the years of training and competition tell the mind that it's time to quit and move on to something else. As we have seen, there are more cases of burn-out in the individual sports like tennis, swimming, and gymnastics because these sports don't have off-season time in which the athlete can rest, regenerate, and pay attention to other activities. Of course, these are sports in which professional training begins at a young age so by the time an athlete is sixteen he or she has already been training and competing for eight or nine years. The psychological burden of this much continuous pressure at such a young age is a principal reason for burnout.

No one seems to be immune to the phenomenon. I've mentioned such high-flying stars as Bjorn Borg and Andrea Jeager who had their careers shortened by burnout and many lesser known athletes have had the same problem. I want to emphasize that the problems are only partly physical. The primary reason is mental.

The best answer to burnout is, as I've said, to start serious training at a later age—the later the better. Another way to prevent overexposure is to reduce training time, especially during the off-season, but not so much that there is a decline in overall conditioning.

I recommend alternative sports—that is, practicing or competing in activities other than the athlete's primary sport. Sports that maintain a high level of aerobic conditioning—basketball, racquetball, handball, golf without a cart—are diverting and fun; and the chance to have fun is important.

On the other hand, I don't recommend that an athlete under eighteen have a summer job unless it too is more fun than work. The young athlete has a job the rest of the year and since they have precious little time to be a child, work for the sake of work will have a negative effect.

△ Drugs, Alcohol, and Sex △

By now, everyone knows that drugs and alcohol are readily available to athletes and that they are often abused by both young and more mature athletes. There is obviously no way to ensure that your youngster will not use and abuse these addictive substances, but a combination of information and education is a step in the right direction.

Over the years I've worked with many athletes who were heavy drug and alcohol abusers. Most of them recovered and continued to play, and play well, but some never did make it back and their careers ended because of their substance abuse. But that isn't the point. We all know that there are criminal penalties for drug use and that going to jail is a possibility, and this also ends a career. But that isn't the point either. In any situation, a sports career (or any other career) is not as important as a life and the lives of these athletes were wasted right along with their careers.

But this argument—that is, saving your life not just your career—does not carry much weight with youngsters because they are not used to thinking in the long term. I've found that the most effective message a parent can deliver to his child about alcohol and drugs is just the opposite—that is, pointing out that these substances can ruin all chances for a professional career. To a youngster the threat of not having a career has more reality, is more immediate and more persuasive than the seemingly abstract idea of saving his life.

The sex issue, though not as life- or career-threatening as drugs and alcohol, is nevertheless another matter that must be brought to the attention of the parents of an aspiring athlete. From a psychological point of view, my experience has confirmed my belief that young people should not have sexual relations before the age of eighteen. I know that makes me sound a bit old-fashioned, but so be it. Regardless of how mature they think they are or how mature they may seem, teenagers are not emotionally equipped to handle the psychological ramifications of intercourse. I realize that the matter can't be legislated, but parental influence can go a long way toward forming a youngster's opinions.

In the sports camps, and later when the athlete is competing professionally, there are pressures and temptations of all kinds and sex is one of those. In tennis, golf, gymnastics, and swimming, there is a good deal of documented evidence of homosexual activity, so the danger signs are clear and as a parent you must observe those signs.

Margaret is a case in point. She is a professional tennis player who came to me when she was sixteen. She had just started on the professional tour at that time and because of financial constraints, her mother wasn't able to travel with her as a chaperone as many mothers do. In the first few weeks she had been absorbed in learning the tour procedures and in her playing, but after about a month she had gotten lonely. Letters and phone calls from her mother weren't enough.

At about the time her loneliness was reaching a crisis point, she was suddenly befriended by one of the established woman pros. Margaret was pleased that someone of that stature was paying attention to her, she liked hanging around with a star, and she was happy to have someone to confide in. The two spent a good deal of time together and it wasn't long before the older woman began making sexual advances toward Margaret. Since the youngster had led a sheltered life and had no real heterosexual experience prior to that time, she had nothing with which to compare what was happening and she was not particularly surprised or shocked by the way she felt. The older woman's approach was sophisticated, warm, and caring, and Margaret found it all very pleasant and rewarding. She was no longer lonely and she had won the approval of other established players by virtue of her relationship with the star. Besides that, her tennis was better than it had ever been.

After a relationship of about a year, the older woman broke off the romance, and that's when Margaret was brought to me by her parents. Margaret was depressed because of her lost love and her parents were upset on two counts: They didn't want to accept the fact that their daughter was a homosexual, and they felt guilty for not having been around to protect her when she needed them most.

I counseled the three of them for several months. During that period I explained that the very real psychological reasons for Margaret's behavior were based in the reality of the situation that occurs when vulnerable children are thrown into an adult environment without supervision. When we finished our sessions, Margaret's parents understood what had happened and Margaret was coming out of her depression with her parents' help.

Of course, heterosexual relationships also develop in these situations and for some of the same reasons—loneliness, inexperience, and experimentation. They are no less difficult to handle, especially when one of the parties is a teenager. As in the case of drugs and alcohol, there is no way to completely protect your youngster from the sexual complications that arise when a teenager lives away from home with adults and without supervision. But it is important to inform your youngster through an honest discussion of the potential problems.

△ The Parent's Role in the Transitional Period and During the Early Professional Career △

The training period for a young athlete may last anywhere from two to five or six years or more depending on the sport and age when training begins. In some cases, all of that time will be spent with private coaches and in various forms of competition. This is particularly true of the individual sports. For some athletes, especially those in team sports, this training period will most likely consist of a combination of private instruction and training camps. Parental support and influence is at its height during these years

Near the end of the training years the athlete and his parents enter a transition period. This occurs, for example, when a young tennis player is about to turn pro or when a college football player enters his senior year. This is the time when the young athlete has reached a level of excellence where he or she is being approached by agents, recruiters, tour directors, business managers, lawyers, sponsors, investors, and con artists, all eager to lead him into his professional career.

During this often rough time of decision-making, parents still have an important role to play because youngsters, as talented as they may be in their sport, are not experienced or mature enough to handle the burgeoning business side of their careers. And preoccupation with matters not directly connected to performance can have a negative psychological impact on performance. So parents must be prepared to help choose their child's advisors.

The agents, the sponsors, and the rest all perform somewhat different roles in the athlete's life. However, it isn't necessary to dissect their roles individually; one set of guidelines will cover most of the issues involved in their choice:

▷ These are powerful people who can be helpful or dangerous to a young athlete's career. Some governing bodies in sports have approved lists of agents, business managers, and the like, but inclusion on this list does not necessarily make that person good for your youngster.

▷ Choose these advisors as carefully as you choose your youngster's coach, and be wary, because many of them are sharp operators who will promise the world.

▷ There are no tests for these jobs and no licenses. Many agents and others have no credentials whatever.

▷ Your child should be comfortable with these advisors, especially the agent, but you must oversee the selection and influence the final choice.

▷ Check references and don't only check with those names given you; do your own checking as well. More than one career has been destroyed by an inexperienced or dishonest advisor.

▷ Be aware that agents are often linked to coaches or specific training programs—that is, the coach recommends the agent and vice versa. This isn't necessarily bad, but you should also look elsewhere for recommendations.

▷ Just as in the coaching situation, the agent who is right for one athlete isn't necessarily right for another. Some don't know how to handle beginning athletes but do fine with established stars; others are just the opposite.

That said, let me assure you that all advisors to athletes are not devious. There are many talented, successful, and honest advisors; but there are also advisors who are quick to take advantage of the unsophisticated and inexperienced athlete and his family and the sports pages regularly carry stories about these unfortunate cases. This is an important choice. Make it with care.

The other issues parents must deal with at this stage include:

1. Relations with the media;

2. Handling temporary setbacks;

3. Continuing to help with psychological and emotional problems;

4. Assistance with and advice about off-season jobs and education;

5. Planning for retirement.

You may think that some of this planning is premature, but it isn't. A career can come to fruition quickly and it can end just as quickly. Preplanning can serve to smooth the emotional ground. I assure you that your time will not be wasted.

Media Relations

Most athletes and many families dream of being the center of media attention. We've all seen the television pictures of a proud family embracing their young athlete after a victory and it's only natural that we put ourselves in that same position. But what may seem like the crowning glory of all your efforts can turn out to be more of a problem than a joy if your youngster becomes a major professional star or Olympic performer, or eventually has a problem that becomes the focus of media attention. It's amazing but true that being on television and radio and in newspapers and magazines may soon become more painful than pleasurable. The right to privacy is as American as Sunday baseball and maintaining privacy in the face of glowing television lights can be difficult and unpleasant.

You have the choice of being protective or open with the media, but it is a decision you should make before it becomes a burning issue. After the fact, under the glare of public attention, there is very little that can be done. You can hire media consultants to handle this facet of your child's professional life, or you can do it yourself. Either way, it is one of those points that should be discussed ahead of time in order to lessen the emotional pressure on the athlete.

Temporary Setbacks

Progress is not necessarily continual. Your child's career may reach a plateau or even go into decline after the professional phase has begun. Such problems as slumps, minor injuries, illness, and conflicts with coaches can all be discussed if the groundwork has been laid for such discussions. Your patience and counsel will be sorely needed at these times. If you think the assistance of a sports psychologist if called for, you should discuss this with your youngster and seek out professional help if agreement is reached on the point.

In general, parents can help best during the professional life of their offspring by continuing to be available for open and frank discussion of problems. This is no easy task, but it falls within the scope of continuing parental responsibility.

Off-Season Jobs and Education

I mentioned earlier that I don't think young professional athletes should have off-season jobs because their full-time, year-around employment is performing in their sport. There are a few exceptions, however, and those fall into the category of low-pressure jobs that are not related to sports, at least to the sport in which the athlete is competing.

I recommend instead that the off-season be used to further the athlete's education as a hedge against serious injury and as preparation for the future. This may include pursuit of an undergraduate or graduate degree, or in some cases, a high school diploma, but it is one of the areas in which parents can, and should, bring pressure to bear. Retirement, whether voluntary or involuntary, is only a jump, a pitch, a tackle, or a back-flip away. Don't forget that careers in team sports last an average of less than five years and it is the rare athlete that competes in any sport past his or her mid-thirties. The time for a second career is never that far off.

△ Life After Sports △

I know it seems odd to talk about life after sports when your young athlete is only entering the sports arena. But unlike retirement from the regular world of work, which usually comes at age sixty or sixty-five, retirement in sports is more often a reality at half that age, an age when most people are moving up in their careers not ending them. Such long-careered stars as Pete Rose in baseball, George Blanda in football, Kareem Abdul Jabbar in basketball, and Jack Nicklaus in golf are the rare exceptions that prove the rule.

The fact is, many athletes who train for specific competitions like the Olympics are finished with active competition when they are still teenagers. Their active careers are over and their whole lives are in front of them. If no plans have been laid, problems lie ahead. In team sports, careers often last longer but only marginally.

Retirement from sports is brought on for several reasons, some voluntary and some forced. There is no mandatory retirement age in sports because there doesn't need to be. Athletes retire when they can no longer compete successfully.

Age and loss of skills The most common reason for retirement is declining ability. Age and the rigors of competition, the years of training, and general wear and tear take their toll and the body loses its ability to perform at the optimum levels needed in professional athletics. For athletes who enjoy long careers the decision to "hang up the spikes" is always difficult but, in the final analysis, that decision is dictated by the body. Depending on the sport and the athlete's job in that sport, some competitors are able to hang on a little longer than others, but by age thirty-five more than 95 percent of all athletes have retired from active competition and by age forty, that percentage is 99.9. In such sports as swimming, gymnastics, and figure skating active competition often ends before age twenty.

Injury. Injuries are a part of sports, particularly contact sports like football and hockey. But all athletes suffer everything from muscle strains to broken bones and all injuries, whether minor or serious, can end careers. An accumulation of minor injuries over a number of years can cause an athlete to decide the pain isn't worth the price. A more serious injury—torn knee ligaments, a broken leg, a back injury, torn rotator cuffs—can, and often does, end an athlete's career by itself—suddenly and prematurely. And though older competitors are somewhat more susceptible, career-ending injuries can come at any time.

Loss of desire or motivation. The loss of desire or motivation can end a career almost as quickly as a serious injury. This reason for retirement is more common today than at any time in the past, primarily for one reason: Athletes are beginning serious training too early and by the time they have reached their early twenties they have already played full careers, suffered a lifetime's worth of injuries, and been under intense pressure for too long.

The Psychological Problems of Retirement

The first feeling an athlete has after retirement for any of the above reasons is one of inadequacy. After years of being on the center of attention from parents, coaches, friends, and the general public—in short, being ahead of the game and on top of the world—he or she is now behind everyone else. After years of having the advantage, the athlete is now at a disadvantage, not the star, not treated specially, not the center of anything.

Along with this inadequate feeling comes a feeling of fear, of not knowing the ropes in the real world. An athlete suddenly finds that his peers are well on the way up the career ladder and he or she is at the bottom. Where the athlete had been in control of events, he or she is no longer in a position to control or dictate much of anything. An athlete's name may get him an job interview but if he doesn't have any other skills, his name alone won't get him that job.

These realities of life can cause frustration, anger, depression, loss of self-esteem, violent mood swings, eating and sleeping disorders, and self-destructive behavior. All of these psychological disorders are treatable if they are recognized for what they are—reactions to a strange and frightening new situation.

Older athletes are better able to deal with their reactions and for the most part won't be relying on their parents for help. But the younger athlete, even up to age twenty-five, who has been nothing but an athlete all his life, will need parental guidance. The parental role here is to try to understand the emotional dynamics involved and to recognize the potential psychological reactions mentioned above for what they are. During this period of trauma, parents need to have the same concern for their youngster that they had during his training and throughout his career. It isn't the time to say, "Grow up," but to pitch in as a family and finish up the job that was begun as a family.

The problems of retirement can't be eliminated, but if some planning has been done for the days after competition—planning that should begin as soon as your youngster's career begins—the problems will be less severe. I can't prescribe the details of that planning, because everyone's situations, abilities, and interests are different, but talking about the realities, keeping up with education, and anticipating the day when competition ends are the first step.

About the Author

In addition to his work as the Executive Director of the Center for Sports Psychology in New York City, Dr. Eric Margenau is a private practitioner who works with parents, coaches and amateur and professional athletes. He is also the consulting sports psychologist for various professional teams. Dr. Margenau writes a New York Daily News column entitled "Psyching It Out" and has appeared frequently on local and network television programs to discuss his work. He is the Editor-in-Chief of a forthcoming book entitled THE ENCYCLOPEDIC HANDBOOK OF PRIVATE PRACTICE, which is the main selection for the Behavioral Science Book Club. The author currently lives in New York City with his wife, Anne, and his children, Danielle and Max.